DR B

Understanding
Hypnosis

A practical guide to the health-giving
benefits of hypnotherapy and self-hypnosis

PIATKUS

Visit the Piatkus website!

Piatkus publishes a wide range of exciting fiction and non-fiction, including books on health, mind body & spirit, sex, self-help, cookery, biography and the paranormal. If you want to:

⌘ read descriptions of our popular

titles

⌘ buy our books over the internet

⌘ take advantage of our special offers

⌘ enter our monthly competition

⌘ learn more about your favourite

Piatkus authors

visit our website at:

www.piatkus.co.uk

Published in the UK in 2000 by
Judy Piatkus (Publishers) Limited
5 Windmill Street
London W1P 1HF
e-mail: info@piatkus.co.uk

A catalogue record for this book is available from the British Library

ISBN 0 7499 2121 8

Page design by Sue Ryall
Edited by Judy Gough

Printed and bound in Great Britain by Bath Press

To Coll,
who heard so much yet said so little

Coll (full name Collingwood) was our ten-year-old Border collie who came from a dogs' home. He was ill-treated as a puppy and had a terror of being left alone. When we went out he would bark incessantly causing neighbours to complain and threaten legal action. In spite of many attempted remedies (including a dog psychiatrist), Coll maintained his barking tendency till the end. He died as I was finishing the last chapter of this book.

He was my constant companion and accompanied me on fishing expeditions, causing havoc by jumping in the water as I was landing a fish. My skill was to try and land Coll and the fish at the same time: too often Coll ended up in the net and the fish swam free. There are many rainbow trout who owe their lives to Coll's presence at the lake.

I took him to work with me three times a week to give my wife (and neighbours) some respite. He listened to all my patients' stories, showing his response by licking the hands of those who burst into tears. He gave a calming and supportive atmosphere to my consulting rooms; any successes I may have had are due in part to Coll's presence.

I do have some concern as to how my practice will fare now that he is gone.

About the Author

Dr Brian Roet trained as a medical doctor in Australia, but now lives in London where he runs a psychotherapy practice. He has been using hypnotherapy for over 20 years to help people manage their emotional health. He is the best-selling author of several books including *All in the Mind?*, *A Safer Place to Cry* and *The Confidence to Be Yourself* (Piatkus) and is regularly featured in the media.

Contents

Acknowledgements

When it comes to Information Technology I am a dinosaur, one of the few people on this planet who have never touched a computer button. I owe my survival to Rekha who has been able to convert my scrawl into a legible manuscript and save me from extinction; for this I am forever indebted.

I would also like to thank Patrick for his literary advice; Georgie for demonstrating the old adage with her illustrations that a picture is worth a thousand words (it would have saved me a lot of time if I had made this a picture book); Katie for her ability to edit my prolonged phrases into succinct sentences; and last but not least, I would like to thank all my patients who have shown me, in their own way, how to understand difficulties and accept limitations.

If you have a past that dissatisfies you, forget it now. Imagine a new story of your life, and believe in it. Concentrate only on those moments in which you achieved what you desired, and this strength will help you to accomplish what you want.

The Fifth Mountain
Paulo Coelho

Introduction

*There are many people to whom the crucial problems of
their lives never get presented in terms they can understand*

I would like to begin by explaining how hypnosis has
become so intertwined with my life and how it could
become so very helpful in yours. I am a 60-year-old doctor
practising hypnosis and psychotherapy in London. My first
40 years were spent in Australia following a pathway of
school, university, medical school and general practice.

In those days we had what were called boozy weekends –
a time away with colleagues to study a specific subject. The
weekend I chose (for no conscious reason) was on hypnosis.
Prior to this I had always regarded hypnosis as mumbo-
jumbo, but during those two days a flicker of interest was
sparked as I saw colleagues in trance, and we discussed the
benefits for general practice.

I forgot about the idea for a month until, for some strange
reason, a patient asked me about hypnosis for her headaches.
I explained I had learnt a little and was willing to try it but
there was no guarantee it would work. She accepted my

proposition and when her headache improved I decided to explore the realms of hypnosis further.

Now, 20 years later, I know much more about the mind and also the role hypnosis can play in resolving many conditions. I use self-hypnosis myself every day to relax and believe it has been of immense help to me in every aspect of my life.

Why am I so intrigued with a technique I originally regarded as mumbo-jumbo? This book contains a summary of my learning over those 20 years. The chapters contain pieces of a jigsaw, still incomplete, as even now we are ignorant about many facets of hypnosis.

What is Hypnosis?

One of my aims in writing this book is to demystify hypnosis. I also hope to give you the confidence to use hypnosis to help you overcome common ailments, phobias and addictions.

After the first hypnosis session patients often say with an embarrassed expression, 'I thought you would swing a gold watch. You just talked to me: I thought it would be very different – I'd look at the swinging watch, go under and wake up cured.' Nothing could be further from the truth as you will find out in the pages ahead.

Hypnosis is in essence a connection between the conscious and unconscious parts of our mind and feels the same as a daydream state – the time when we have just woken up and just before we go to sleep. It has been found that this state provides many resources unavailable in the conscious state alone.

I would like to make two important points at this stage:

the first is the distinction between medical hypnosis, or hypnotherapy, which is used to help resolve medical problems, and stage hypnosis which is used for entertainment. These two are as different as driving a Mini about London and driving a Ferrari in a Formula One Grand Prix race. They are both driving but what a difference!

The second point is that hypnotherapy is the safest form of therapy I know. In all the 20 years I have been practising and after treating many thousands of patients there has not been one case of anyone being harmed by hypnosis.

Hypnotherapy and Conventional Medicine

When I graduated in Australia, it was forbidden to refer patients to alternative therapists as we risked being struck off the medical register. Fortunately, the general attitude to complementary therapies such as osteopathy or acupuncture has relaxed a great deal over the years and although English people, perhaps due to their reserved nature, have found hypnotherapy more difficult to accept than people in other countries such as Australia or America, it has in recent times become much more acceptable both to the medical profession and general public. It is now recognised that there is more to the restoration of health than tablets or operations and that these therapies can help when medical treatment fails.

The results of research into the benefits of hypnotherapy are being published in medical journals. These articles are presented in a scientific manner with well-ordered trials showing how hypnotherapy can cure conditions such as irritable bowel syndrome, a condition previously in the domain of the gastroenterologists.

Hypnosis is not a panacea to cure all ills. It is a complementary therapy working alongside medical practice. In that way the patient receives the best attention from two different points of view. It is important that the GP forms a central link during the patient's treatment so that different people are not unaware of others' involvement. The busy GP sees many patients whose symptoms originate in the mind. As these patients are time consuming and keep returning, more and more practices are employing counsellors, psychotherapists and hypnotherapists.

The Trance State

Hypnotherapy is a connection of two words – hypnosis and therapy. Hypnosis itself is not a treatment (apart from being relaxing), but is needed to perform the treatment (the therapy). Many people confuse the two and focus on the hypnosis rather than the therapy. The purpose is to use the benefit of the trance state, where conscious and unconscious minds are communicating, to aid therapy. The role of the hypnotherapist is to use his skills and make suggestions to help patients solve their problems (physical or psychological) while in this trance state. During a session the aim is to:

- Help you to relax.
- Enable you to communicate with your unconscious and resolve your problem.
- Teach you about yourself.
- Give you an improved, up-to-date perspective.
- Help connect your thoughts and feelings.

Achieving these aims requires expertise from the therapist and a willingness to co-operate from the patient. It is not someone doing something to someone else just as a driving instructor is not making the learner drive – he is teaching, supporting, providing ways and means to practise what is taught, being a guide until the learner can drive alone. So it is with hypnotherapy. The expertise of the therapist is not so much how to hypnotise someone – that is relatively easy – it is how to make use of the trance state to resolve the patient's problem.

The methods of achieving this state are many and varied and depend on the preference of the therapist; they may either be directive where the therapist takes the role of an authority figure directing the patient to make choices, or indirect where more subtle messages are given avoiding conscious resistance.

Why Use Hypnosis?

Hypnosis explores the mind and its role in disease. Many people realise their mind may be responsible for their complaint and more and more of them are seeking hypnotherapy as a way to resolve the problem. It is a very safe form of therapy which uses no medicines, with their potential side-effects, and does not carry the same risks as an operation. It aims to treat the problem rather than to deaden it with tablets and this is making it increasingly popular with patients who see the benefits of such an approach.

Spending time with a patient is one of the most valuable ways a doctor or therapist can be of help. Attentive listening has been shown to be a major factor in the resolution of many symptoms – listening to both the conscious and unconscious has even more benefit and allows us to see a clearer, more balanced picture of what is happening when symptoms develop.

Imagine you are in a room and an unpleasant smell is disturbing your concentration. You search the room but cannot find the cause, so you hope it will go away by itself. The next day the smell is still there and you try to put it to the back of your mind but it keeps interfering with your enjoyment of the day. You search some more but still without success. At night you begin to worry that the smell will still be there in the morning and your sleep is disturbed. This situation continues, distracting you and altering your personality so that friends comment on the change.

Eventually you decide to search outside the room. Opening a cupboard under the stairs you discover some food left over from a picnic. Immediately you feel better, you are in control again. After a few days the smell has completely gone and you return to your former self.

Our problems are often similar to the unpleasant smell; they prevent us from being ourselves and achieving our real potential. We tend to search for solutions in places we know in spite of the fact that we are not achieving results. Hypnosis helps us 'look under the stairs' to remove the cause of our problem. It is in essence a way of learning about ourselves without conflict or confrontation.

Self-hypnosis

It has been said that all hypnosis is self-hypnosis and that the therapist merely acts as a catalyst. In essence self-hypnosis means putting yourself in a trance. This generally consists of having quiet undisturbed time, focusing intently (either inwardly or on an object) and allowing yourself to drift down to a deep level of relaxation by talking to yourself in a positive and repetitious way. It has been shown that achieving this deep state of relaxation has many benefits. It allows you a different perspective on your problems; enables you to communicate with your unconscious; reduces pain, stress and anxiety; rebuilds lost energy; and helps you learn about yourself so you can achieve your full potential.

How to Use This Book

In order for this to be a self-help book, you will need to employ the text to help you, and in so doing make changes to some aspects of your life – your lifestyle, your attitude, your thinking, your belief system, the way your past affects you and so on. The benefits you will achieve are related to how you digest some of the facts you read. It is possible to keep them 'out there' as 'interesting but not relevant to me', or you can apply different chapters to your own personal situation.

Read the book one chapter at a time giving yourself time to digest it. Like a meal, you don't go from one plate of food to the next without a break and you allow time between lunch and dinner to digest and enjoy what you have taken in. The chapters are set out in an organised way leading you through the process of learning about hypnosis: what it is, the different forms of hypnosis, how to use self-hypnosis, what to expect in a consultation and how to deal with a number of common problems. Case histories will illustrate the points made and the techniques involved. You can use these to focus on something that triggers off a personal response: 'I do that', 'I feel just like she did', 'That's the way I react', and use this knowledge to treat yourself.

Make a commitment to practise self-hypnosis, firstly for relaxation and then for specific aims. Regard your unconscious as a friend you would like to know better so it can help you in future situations.

Throughout this book to avoid confusion of the 'he/she' notation, I will use 'he' to denote an abstract person. Also I choose to use 'patient' rather than 'client' because of my medical background.

And lastly I would like to repeat that hypnotherapy has been used for hundreds of years, it is natural, safe and works for many conditions. The more you learn about it the more benefit you will gain from its use. It is not a cure-all but can be a major factor in restoring balance to lives that are pressurised, stressful and over-committed.

As I have already said it has been a great friend and benefactor for me and I hope in some way it will be for you too.

PART I

Learning About Hypnosis

1

What is Hypnosis?

Many ideas grow better when transplanted into another mind than in the one where they originated

Oliver Wendell Holmes

If ever there was a word that has caused the imagination to run wild with vivid pictures, it is hypnosis. Unfortunately most of these pictures are incorrect when it comes to medical hypnosis or hypnotherapy. Even the word itself is incorrect; it is derived from Hypnos, the Greek God of Sleep, but it is not sleep – it is a trance state.

Historically hypnosis has been used since Egyptian times – there are hieroglyphs in the Tomb of Isis showing worshippers experiencing hypnotic states. The term 'hypnosis' was coined by Dr James Braid, a Scottish physician, who lived from 1785–1860. It gained popularity in India in 1850 when a surgeon, James Esdaile, performed many operations including amputations, using hypnosis as the sole anaesthetic. Today it is used by many therapists around the world to help with stress, anxiety, pain relief, phobias or just deep relaxation.

One of the main difficulties which has prevented

hypnosis becoming more popular is people's fear due to false information that has gathered over time. I asked a number of people what they thought hypnosis would do for them if they went to see a hypnotherapist:

- 'I'd never go, I'd lose control.'
- 'I'm frightened I'd never wake up.'
- 'I'm sure I'd go to sleep and wake up with the problem solved.'
- 'It would open up a can of worms and I'd never be the same.'
- 'The hypnotist would make me do things I didn't want to.'

All of these views are incorrect. The surprising thing is that we go in and out of a trance many times a day. Many problems are maintained because we hypnotise ourselves with incorrect beliefs.

Hypnosis is a natural phenomenon that occurs in a cyclical rhythm throughout the day. It is a completely different state from sleep and has very different actions on the mind and body. To understand what I mean we need to look at the three components running our lives:

1. **Our conscious mind** is the part that works within our awareness. We have control, we know what is happening and make decisions of our own choice.

2. **Our unconscious mind** consists of all of our experiences and memories. We do not have control of thoughts or behaviour arising from this part.

3. **Our feelings** and emotions are represented in different parts of our body and these too are beyond our control

– they respond to thoughts from the conscious and unconscious parts and may or may not be appropriate.

Whilst we are awake we fluctuate between the conscious and unconscious minds and are influenced by both; often the unconscious is helpful whilst at other times its actions are out of date and unsuitable. If we have psychological problems relating to past experiences then the unconscious mind is causing those problems. Hypnosis is useful in learning about the role this part of our mind is playing.

One definition of hypnotherapy is: 'Communicating with the unconscious and updating it.' Our past creates many beliefs that we hold. Hypnosis can be very useful in analysing these beliefs and assessing whether we wish to continue them for the rest of our lives.

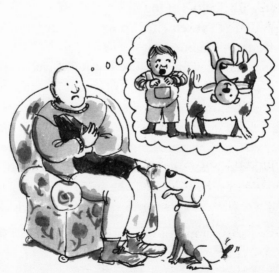

If we have psychological problems relating to past experiences then the unconscious mind is causing these problems.

Joanne is 45. She has a lonely life. She goes to work as a secretary then goes home to her flat and budgerigar. She has few friends and feels low most of the time.

At school in London, Joanne was picked on and ostracised because she had a Yorkshire accent. The other girls in the class kept teasing and bullying her. As this continued for some years Joanne became self-conscious, shy and introverted. She learnt there was something terribly wrong with her, what other reason could there be for the awful treatment she received.

When she left school she maintained her hibernation and apart from a secretarial course kept to herself. Life seemed to have passed her by.

Joanne came to see me because she was not sleeping properly. She was having nightmares where she was chased by evil women or animals; she was exhausted and having difficulty coping.

When I asked her how she got on with her workmates she burst into tears.

'No one likes me because I'm repulsive.'

I was surprised at the comment because she was a normal, healthy-looking woman. In spite of my contradicting her she repeated that it was obvious that was the way she was and I was making it worse by being patronising.

Due to her experience in childhood, Joanne's unconscious had decided she must be repulsive and this opinion was very strong in spite of the obvious evidence to the contrary.

It took many months of hypnotherapy for Joanne's unconscious to realise the fault was that the children in the school were being mean and nasty to a perfectly normal girl whose only 'fault' was to have a Yorkshire accent.

In order to learn more about hypnosis we need to learn about the conscious and unconscious minds and the feelings resulting from them. Future chapters will discuss these in further detail.

Hypnosis makes use of the natural phenomenon of changing from conscious to unconscious states that is constantly happening during the day. When we say we are 'absent-minded', we mean our conscious mind is absent which implies our unconscious mind is present. When we daydream, we 'go off' somewhere and are 'brought back' to our conscious awareness by some noise or remark. This daydream state is very similar to the one we feel during hypnosis. It is the state we are in just before we go to sleep and on waking in the morning. It is called an 'altered state' or 'trance'.

When we drive, due to the routine, we often go into a trance. Our conscious minds are focused on some problem while the unconscious does the driving. Often we arrive home completely unaware of the journey. This is even more so with the modern motorist using a mobile phone at the same time. The mind is divided into the driver, listener, talker and thinker.

Hypnosis is the technique used to communicate with different parts of the kaleidoscope we call the mind. By inducing a 'trance' or 'altered state' the hypnotherapist can talk to the unconscious without the conscious blocking communication. A simple example:

Joe is terrified of going on a bus. His unconscious gives him panic attacks if he attempts to board one.

Telling Joe it is safe to travel by bus would not resolve his problem because it radiates from his unconscious mind. Using hypnosis we can influence this part of Joe's mind so it, like his conscious mind, can be aware of the real facts.

It is likely that Joe has developed his phobia from a past experience, when he was not in control, which has been stored in his unconscious. This means he is unable to use his rational thinking. By bypassing the conscious and communicating with the unconscious in a trance we can alter his perspective so that the reaction to buses is based on up-to-date facts rather than early memories.

A simplistic model of the mind that I find useful is the 'open door'. Imagine two rooms with a door between: if we call one conscious and the other unconscious then the door between enables communication. Normally the door is closed and the conscious room is in control. When our critical faculties are diminished the door opens. This occurs in childhood or when an intense emotion is felt such as fear, anxiety, sadness, guilt, etc. The open door allows the experience to penetrate the second room and a mechanism is set up to deal with any similar situations in the future. The system then remains dormant until it is triggered by something that bears a similarity to the initiating experience. When this trigger occurs the door opens and the reactionary mechanism is brought into play, the conscious mind being powerless to intervene.

The conscious and unconscious work on different levels and influence us in different ways. Often these influences are in conflict as the following example shows.

A man gets stuck in a lift. The lights fail and he is left in darkness. His critical faculties are overcome with fear, thoughts of death and feelings of panic. Some time later, when the lift is repaired, he is able to continue his day

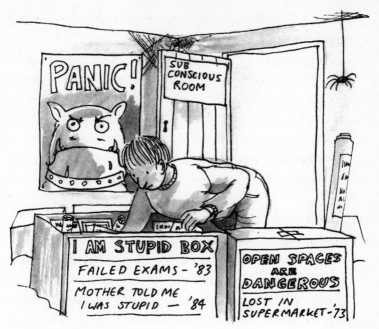

The Subconscious Room

normally, perhaps telling his friends about the frightening experience.

But the door has been opened and the message, 'If you go in a lift you will die', forced into the unconscious. It reacts by devising a method 'to save his life' and preventing him going into a lift by causing panic attacks whenever he approaches one.

Hypnosis is helpful as it, too, is able to open the door and re-educate the unconscious with more suitable facts and figures than the bare statement 'lifts kill'. This process enables new information, closer to reality, to be directed to the unconscious so that the defensive mechanism of panic attacks can be reduced.

The role of hypnosis is to allow the transfer of knowledge between the conscious and unconscious. In the case of the man who was stuck in a lift he would be taught to go into a trance, and in this more suggestible state, information would be given to him by the therapist to enable the unconscious mind to let go of the fear. The therapist may point out that many millions of people travel safely in lifts; he has been in lifts for many years without mishap; nothing untoward happened when the lift was stuck; the risk involved is minimal. All these facts will be more readily accepted in the trance state than in the normal alert state of mind.

It is imperative that the door between the two minds is opened, otherwise we remain stuck in the conscious and can use only logic and analysis to help. As the unconscious generally works with feelings it is important that resolution is via the mediation of feelings too.

The majority of patients who seek help do so for feelings, emotions causing pain, suffering and limitations. It can be assumed that when people seek hypnosis they have already tried consciously to do everything they can, so it would be futile to use the 'pull your socks up' and 'get on with it' approach. We utilise hypnosis to get in touch with our feelings, and in doing so we are able to interact with the unconscious and unlock the mechanism causing the problem. This imaginary door will not be battered down as unconscious resistance is very strong. It needs to be treated gently, subtly, with respect, so that the exchange of information and experience progresses with trust and negotiation.

When used in therapy, hypnosis is the creating of an altered state (trance), so that the unconscious can help the patient solve a problem that he is unable to solve in the conscious state. The therapist helps him gain access to resources he has but doesn't realise he has.

There is a 'society for lost knowledge'. It consists of a group of people endeavouring to rediscover things we once knew, such as how the pyramids were built and Stonehenge was constructed. Hypnosis is like this society. The therapist is trying to help us gain access to the knowledge and ability we do not know we have stored away in the unconscious.

Hypnosis is a natural everyday phenomenon used to communicate with the unconscious and update it, so that the patients' own resources can be utilised to solve their problems.

2

Why Hypnosis?

Hypnosis helps you relax deeply and re-organise your thoughts, feelings and attitudes. This has a powerful influence on self-confidence and stress reduction.

Brian Roet

Hypnosis, when used clinically to treat patients, is called 'hypnotherapy' and the therapist needs to be trained in counselling, psychotherapy and hypnosis. The consultation consists mainly of psychotherapy in both conscious and trance states – hypnosis being a tool to aid therapy. A suitable metaphor may be a door-lock that is stuck, and the door will not open. Some intervention is necessary so a locksmith with knowledge of that particular mechanism is brought in to repair and open the door. In the same way hypnosis is the few drops of oil that may make all the difference.

Why choose hypnosis instead of the multitude of other therapies available today? I asked a number of patients that very question. Some of the replies were:

- 'I knew my problem was in my mind; I came because hypnosis helps unravel problems of the mind.'

- 'I was fed up with taking tablets and yet more tablets. The side-effects were becoming worse than the problem.'
- 'I am so tense I know I need to relax.'
- 'I need to understand what is going on in my head. I feel my mind is my worst enemy.'
- 'I've tried everything else and this is my last hope.'
- 'I want treatment where I am involved but I don't want to spend years in analysis.'
- 'I believe I am only working at a very superficial level. I know by my dreams and difficulty with sleeping something is going on at a deeper level and I want to explore this.'

Hypnosis is not therapeutic by itself. It does provide focused attention, relaxation, a quiet time and a state of 'being' rather than 'trying'; this gives a balance to the hectic pace of everyday life. It is very similar to meditation and not tailored to any specific needs or problems.

Hypnotherapy is a much more complex process and there are many factors involved in each consultation:

1. Time devoted solely to the patient and their needs.
2. Support, understanding and attentive listening from the therapist.
3. Interpretations, reflections and improved perspective of the patient's belief systems and attitudes.
4. Utilisation of the many properties of hypnosis to achieve the patient's aims. The basic aims of hypnotherapy are: to help the patient understand how he is maintaining his problem; to provide techniques to overcome his problem; and, if it is suitable, to teach him self-hypnosis so he can make use of the benefits of the trance state to resolve his problem.

During hypnotherapy the patient learns a great deal about ways he has been maintaining his problem, both on a conscious and unconscious level. Patterns of behaviour (often stemming from childhood) are explored from an adult perspective and the conflict between thinking and feeling examined. Generally problems involve emotions that are inappropriate and excessive for the situation concerned.

A patient seeking help will not always be advised to use hypnosis when counselling and psychotherapy on a conscious level may be the best way to achieve a solution. I am wary of patients who request 'hypnosis to fix my problem' as they generally have a belief that the therapist will 'fix them' while they sit there with their eyes closed. It should be repeated that hypnosis is a tool that is a useful adjunct to therapy. Just as drops of oil alone will not open the door, so it is with hypnosis. The sharing, listening, exploring, interpreting, supporting and guiding are all necessary to turn the handle and open the door to freedom from the symptom.

The therapist regards symptoms as messages that need understanding and resolving. Out-of-date and inappropriate emotions which are still present in the unconscious are the most common cause of symptoms. Exploring the symptom will lead to identifying these emotions so they can be expressed and released, thus resolving the conflict and removing the symptom.

The medical profession has a view that a symptom is a problem that needs fixing with a tablet. This approach is vastly different from the 'symptoms as messages' view of the therapist. Tablets may stop the symptom temporarily but as the underlying conflict has not been addressed it may well return.

Years ago one of the criticisms was that if a symptom is removed by hypnosis another will take its place. This was called 'symptom substitution', but research over the last ten years has shown this is not the case except in some special conditions such as hysterical personality.

Tapping the Unconscious

The conscious mind contains many facts and attitudes, so does the unconscious. Returning to the image of two rooms – representing the conscious and the unconscious – and a door between the two allowing information to travel both ways, 'trying' closes the door; going into a 'being' – accepting what is happening – state allows the door to open. We all have experience of trying to remember a name that is on the tip of our tongue – the harder we try the further the name moves away. When we stop trying and think of something else, it reappears. This is one way hypnotherapy works. By directing a patient into the trance state many things happen, one of which is that the door opens and we gain access to our unconscious strengths.

Jenny received £3,000 from the sale of some furniture. She decided to buy a car and hid the money in the meantime. It took three months to find the right car, and then she had forgotten where she had hidden the money. She searched her flat from top to bottom many times, to no avail. She asked friends and family to help; still no money. She worried, fretted, tossed and turned at night but the hiding place remained a secret. After another three months she was desperate, and came to me to see if hypnosis could unlock her memory. She had no great faith in the idea but was prepared to try anything.

Jenny was a deep subject and easily went into a trance.

I talked to her about her unconscious having the answer and by relaxing and allowing the door to open she would realise where the hiding place was.

A week later she rang to say she had a dream that it was under her daughter's mattress and there it was. By teaching her to relax and stop worrying, the answer appeared in a dream created by the unconscious.

Hypnosis as a Natural State

The trance, as already said, is a naturally occurring state of mind described as a meditative, altered or daydream state – a deeply relaxing 'being' state, compared with the doing state we are in most of the day. A simplified view is that we go up and down constantly between conscious awareness and an altered state. Each has its benefits and by fluctuating between the two we gain the best of both worlds.

Ernest Rossi, an American psychologist studying the mind's activities, found that if there is no pressure to do anything during the day, we remain in a conscious state for 90 minutes then move into a trance state for 20 minutes in a repetitive pattern. He called this process 'ultradian rhythm' and found it applied to everyone who was pressure free and allowed to do what they want. He also found it applied to animals. His theory is that we are pressurised by modern life to stay in the conscious state and to miss out on the benefits and healing power of the trance state.

Self-hypnosis is one way of spending time in an altered state of mind and in his book, *The Twenty-Minute Break*, (Palisades Gateway, 1991) Rossi points out how beneficial this relaxing time is to achieving our full potential. By using 'trance time' daily we provide an essential ingredient that nature intended.

Safety

Due to the impact of stage-hypnosis many people believe it is unsafe to be hypnotised. The belief that you will be put under a spell by some Svengali figure is so far from the truth that it is laughable. Instead of being powerful to the extent that it takes control, my concern about hypnosis is that it is often not powerful enough to cause important changes. The mind has a basic resistance to being changed by outside influences. If I saw a patient who had a fear of flying, hypnotised him and told him his fear would go away, it would have little effect. The causes for his fear would not have been addressed and the reason not to fly would still be present. Unconscious resistance would ensure I did not change his mind by this method.

The process by which patients make changes is complex and involves many factors:

1. Motivation.
2. Trust in the therapist.
3. A willingness to change.
4. Time and effort by the patient.
5. The trance state.
6. Hypnotic techniques by the therapist.
7. The passage of time.
8. Resolution of unconscious conflicts.

Unless most of these components are addressed, change will not occur.

It is important to realise 'the therapist is on your side, working with you to achieve your aims'. You and the therapist work together as a team to achieve what you want. This means that the session should not be frightening or threatening, but comfortable, supporting and enlightening.

Hypnotherapy is very safe. It is important that you find a therapist who suits your needs and is on your wavelength. There are no risks with hypnosis and side-effects are minimal. You may feel a little tired after a session; you may have a slight headache indicating activity in a part of your mind not normally accessible. This is similar to doing physical exercise and feeling muscle aches afterwards.

Some people are concerned they may 'open a can of worms' if they explore past experiences with hypnosis. With a competent therapist, going at your own pace, it is unlikely that this will cause problems. The therapist may well be able to make use of any problems and convert them into opportunities for you to learn how past experiences play a role in your present attitudes. Generally the unconscious will release only memories that you can cope with, as mechanisms of protection are very strong indeed.

Sometimes people tell me things in a trance and forget them completely when they return to the conscious state. In this way the unconscious can communicate with me and use amnesia to prevent disturbance of the conscious mind.

How Do You Choose Your Therapist?

This is an important question but not an easy one to answer. It applies to any form of help you are seeking. How do you choose your doctor, dentist, electrician, plumber?

The most reliable way is by personal reference from someone who has seen a therapist and been helped. The first port of call should be your general practitioner, as he knows you and your problem, and will be able to refer you to a suitable hypnotherapist if you request one.

Recommendation from a friend is often helpful, especially if they have seen the therapist themselves. It must be taken into account that we have different needs and therapists may suit some people but not others. Societies of hypnosis (see p. 270) will send the names of therapists practising hypnosis in your area.

Before you make an appointment ask as many questions of the therapist as you need to. Enquire about his training, societies he belongs to, how many sessions it will take (this is often difficult without an actual consultation), fees and length of consultation. It is also worth getting recommendations from previous patients.

When you first see the therapist be aware of your intuition, your gut reaction (see p. 84). As I have said, you and the therapist are a team working together to solve your problem. You need to feel confident and positive that your therapist is the right person to help you. If you do not feel comfortable, discuss your feelings with him; remember he is on your side, and if the feeling is not resolved it may be better to seek help elsewhere. It is really important that you trust and believe in your therapist so that your problems can be explored and solved.

As you can see from this chapter 'Why Hypnosis?' is not a simple question to answer. Hypnotherapy has many advantages in that it is natural, safe, with few side-effects and helps you understand yourself. When you find a therapist who suits your needs, all these advantages can be brought into play to resolve your problem.

3

Techniques

All our interior world is reality – and that perhaps more so than our external world.

Marc Chagall

The Trance State

Some doctors believe that many illnesses occur because our busy lives prevent us going into a trance as nature intended (see p. 16). Hypnotherapy makes use of this trance to help you help yourself. Being deeply relaxed, the mind is more receptive to suggestions. These suggestions are put to you by the therapist in a calm, relaxed and monotonous voice. He does this so as not to bring you back to your conscious state which would occur with animated conversation.

It is understandable that people have doubts and fears about a trance because it is the 'unknown'. Most of these are unfounded but should be answered by the therapist.

'Doctor, how will I know if I'm hypnotised?' is a common question when people come for help. It is not an easy question to answer as, while some people are unaware that they are in a trance, others feel it very strongly. They may find they just feel very deeply, very pleasantly relaxed. When they come back to the room and open their eyes they may believe much more time has elapsed than it actually has. This is called time distortion; often an hour seems like ten minutes, and it is as if there is 'mind time' and 'clock time'. Sometimes people have different sensations – heaviness, lightness, tingling, anaesthesia – or they are aware of being in a dream-like state without the need to be in control. They may recall things they haven't thought of for years. They may go back to previous experiences, 'regression', and undergo them again, just as they happened.

Emotions are frequently released during a trance – tears, laughter, anger – as patients release feelings that have been repressed. A great relief is often felt as this occurs.

Trance Capacity

We all have what is called a 'trance capacity' – the ability to go into a trance. It is unrelated to intelligence or strength of mind. Some people are capable of going into a deep trance, others into a light one and some may not respond at all to the techniques of the hypnotherapist.

'I'm sure I can't be hypnotised', is another comment I hear very often. I find it strange that someone coming to see me for hypnotherapy makes such a statement. The ability to be hypnotised depends on:

1. Your basic trance capacity.
2. Your trust in the therapist.
3. Your willingness to 'let go' and allow what happens to happen.

4. Your ability to suspend judgement, reduce analysis and relinquish the need to be in control.
5. The personality and abilities of the therapist.

We can lessen our ability to go into a trance by not trusting the therapist, being fearful of what may be said, being resistant for some reason, needing to be in control or expecting more of hypnosis than actually occurs.

The trance state is essentially a very relaxing one. It is a state of 'letting go' and allowing all the pressures of life to fade into the distance while focusing on the issue at hand. In essence it is a state where you are intensely focused on internal thoughts or feelings so that external disturbances are ignored. Many people enjoy it so much they say, 'I really didn't want to come back into the room it was so peaceful and calm.'

In Australia my consulting rooms were on a main road. One day I was hypnotising a woman and suggesting she relax and imagine she was lying in the sun on a beautiful desert island. She sat very quietly focusing on her island, deeply involved in the relaxation and peace.

Suddenly there was a terrific crash outside, followed by the sound of breaking glass and rolling hub-caps. I was concerned both for the people in the crash and also how the noise would affect my patient. However, she remained motionless with her face calm and focused. When she came out of the trance I asked her about her experience.

'It was wonderful, calm and relaxing. My island was beautiful. I was disturbed for a little while by a noisy boat but that passed by and I was able to relax again.'

This woman was able to integrate the outside noise into her inner world and keep it at a distance from her focus on calmness and relaxation.

My partner, who was working in another room, looked after those involved in the accident and luckily no one was seriously hurt.

You do *not* need to make your mind go blank; letting your thoughts drift by, like fluffy white clouds, allows you to achieve calmness and the ability to drift into a trance. There are three parts to a trance: induction, utilisation and coming out of a trance.

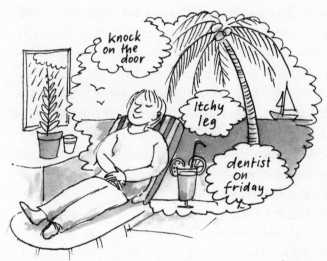

Letting your thoughts drift by, like fluffy clouds, allows you to achieve calmness and the ability to drift into a trance.

Induction

The induction is the process of guiding you from the conscious, alert, rational state of mind into the internally focused emotional state of a trance.

There are numerous in which induction occurs. The first step is to *focus* on something either external (an object) or internal (a thought).

While this focus is maintained – occupying the conscious mind – the therapist talks in a monotonous voice to help you relax, let go and float into unconscious thinking and feeling. Often tears are shed as people drift into an emotional state.

The methods used by different therapists vary considerably – some go through progressive relaxation, others count backwards from 100, others tell stories or repeat calming words – all are used to guide you into the deeply relaxed state called trance.

It may be that several sessions are required to help you achieve your trance capacity or it may be that you are able to let go in the first session and feel the deeply relaxing sensation that accompanies this state. There are often many concerns that are raised in the initial sessions: 'Is it working, I don't feel any different?', 'I'm sure I could open my eyes if I tried', 'I wonder what the therapist is doing now?', 'My arms are getting heavy, I hope I don't stay this way'.

In time and with experience these worries diminish. Each time you go into a trance you will realise how normal, comfortable and natural it is. Practising self-hypnosis at home (see Chapter 5) will demonstrate that it is something very worthwhile to balance the tensions and pressures of everyday life.

As a therapist I can see if the patient sitting opposite me is in a trance in response to my induction. They are very still; their eyes may move behind their eyelids; they have the intense appearance of being focused; their breathing is even and regular; small tears may appear in the corners of their eyes; and at the end of the trance they will say it seemed shorter than it actually was.

But the person in a trance may be unaware of all these phenomena and also have doubts as to what actually happened, if anything at all. Again I would like to repeat that the aim is to *get better* not to be hypnotised, so if you feel you weren't hypnotised and your condition improves that is a satisfactory outcome.

Initially, some of the feelings of going into a trance relate to the fact that there are very few situations in life where you sit opposite a stranger with your eyes closed. Try it with a friend and notice all the emotions that arise – 'What is he thinking?', 'How do I look?', 'Do I feel out of control?', 'I want to open my eyes and see what is happening.'

You may also feel any or all of the following: heaviness, lightness, tingling, cold, light-headedness, flashbacks of experiences, emotions of all varieties, calmness, out-of-body sensations and numbness. All return to normal when you come out of the trance.

Techniques to Put Yourself Into a Trance

There are many ways to change from the conscious state to the trance state. They all involve quiet, undisturbed time – 20 minutes once or twice a day.

A visualising technique involving levels of the mind

1. Close your eyes and take a minute or two to focus internally, allowing time for your active attitude to move to a passive one.

2. Focus on your breathing; as you breathe out allow yourself to float down for ten breaths.

3. Imagine your mind having many levels, the top one being your conscious, alert state, and the bottom one a deep sleep.

4. Move down one level from the top one. Stay at this first level feeling more relaxed and explore what is present there, noticing any way this differs from the level above.

5. When you are ready, drift down to the next level and learn what is present there. Take as long as you want; there is no hurry and you don't have to explore any more levels than you wish.

6. Over the remaining minutes either explore other levels, becoming more relaxed with each one, or remain on a level that feels comfortable so you can learn more about it.

7. When you feel ready to finish the trance, focus on your in-breaths and rise up through the levels until you reach the top one and then open your eyes.

Different people have various ways of visualising these levels and utilising them to discover more about themselves.

Michael came to see me to learn about self-hypnosis. He had heard that it was very helpful and had read a book about it. He had no specific problem but wished to learn more about himself. I decided to use the different level technique to start Michael on his journey.

He sat quietly exploring the different levels and making a few remarks about his findings. For Michael his trance revealed the following:

'The top level is like an office, very busy with people rushing around, computers and telephones. It feels stressful and I notice my neck is tense at this level. I used an escalator to go down the levels. The next level down is like a gym. People are working at exercise machines. It is much quieter and less hectic but a lot of intensity is there. I would like to do some exercises but I think I'll explore further.

'The next level is more like a lounge, there is no one else here, it is quiet and some music is playing. I sit in a comfortable chair and relax. I think I'll stay here as it feels really good.'

When Michael came out of the trance he was a little surprised.

'I didn't realise my imagination was so good. I knew somehow there were many more levels but I just didn't want to leave the lounge.'

People have many and varied 'safe places' that they imagine. One man enjoyed being in a concrete bunker with no windows; another created a secluded garden that no one could enter without his permission; many people choose their childhood bedroom, others a home they desire in the future. Some choose to be on their own; others want an armed guard; others still want their partner or pet to be with them in the safe place.

A safe place

1. Close your eyes and focus on your breathing.

2. Take a little while to float down with each out-breath, becoming more relaxed each time you breathe out.

3. When you feel ready, imagine a safe place – it may be somewhere you have been or somewhere you would like to be. It may be a real place or one you construct yourself.

4. Your safe place can be anything you want and it can contain anything you wish. It may be a room, a field, a beach, a house and you can be with many people or alone. The only requirement is that you really feel safe and confident.

5. Go into your safe place and enjoy the feeling there. You may decide just to stay with this feeling or view some aspect of your life from the safety of this place.

6. The feelings to focus on while you are in your safe place are: safety, comfort, confidence and control.

7. Remain there as long as you wish and be aware you can re-create this place any time you need to.

8. When you are ready, leave and return to the room.

Different parts of the body, and particularly the heart, may be used to contain the safe place so you can go there whenever you wish.

One of the main points is that it is not what you believe is 'correct' or what you 'should' choose but that it is your choice, and the feeling of safety and confidence is an essential ingredient. Though each time you go into a trance may be different, it is entirely dependent on your desire and creativity.

Eye-roll technique

1. Sit or lie with your head supported.

2. Look up towards your forehead, straining your eyes a little.

3. Take a deep breath in and hold it.

4. After five seconds slowly let your breath out and allow your eyelids to close.

5. Hold your out-breath for five seconds then breathe in deeply, open your eyes and look up again.

6. Hold the in-breath for five seconds then breathe out, slowly closing your eyes a second time.

7. Hold your out-breath again for five seconds then breathe in, open your eyes and look up for five seconds.

8. Close your eyes slowly as you breathe out and leave them closed as you focus on your out-breaths, floating down with each one.

9. Stay in this deeply relaxed state being aware of the different sensations that you feel. You will drift and float in a trance, allowing thoughts to come and go. The outside world will seem far away.

10. When you are ready after 15–20 minutes, focus on your in-breaths, rise up to the conscious state and open your eyes.

This technique is a very rapid way to go into a trance. It was developed by Dr Herbert Spiegel, an American psychiatrist who noticed that some very deeply hypnotic subjects rolled up their eyes as they went into a trance. Many people use this technique to block out the outside world – when travelling on the underground or on a plane – and find it a really refreshing way to use the journey time.

Trance Utilisation

This is the reason for hypnotherapy. The therapist uses the trance to provide a state of mind where therapy will be more effective. If therapeutic suggestions are made at the conscious level they will be blocked by logical, rational thought.

'I am terrified of flying, can you help me, doctor?'
'Yes. Here are the statistics that show how safe it is to fly.'

This advice is unlikely to be of any help at all as the communication is taking place on a conscious level. Using a trance, and providing access to resources that the patient already possesses in other areas, may well resolve the problem.

To help guide people into a trance the therapist uses a monotonous tone and words that are unlikely to stimulate a return to the conscious state. In this way the patient can drift into the daydream state and be receptive to any positive suggestions used in the therapy.

By continuing to explore ways and means of achieving an improved attitude and pathways to a solution, the patient is being positively 'brainwashed' by a supportive therapist to overcome the negative 'brainwashing' that has caused the problem. This negative brainwashing, whether by parents, teachers or school children, may have occurred in childhood, and is being maintained by habit and repetition in the unconscious.

As all living things are resistant to change, there are many barriers to deny or avoid suggestions made to facilitate change. The skill of the therapist is to use the trance and his therapeutic language to overcome these barriers and alter negative belief systems that are causing the problem.

Geoff, a 30-year-old mechanic came to see me because of extreme outbursts of uncontrollable temper causing problems at work – he had smashed the office telephone a week before and was worried he might lose his job. He had also hit Freda, his girlfriend, and she, understandably, wanted to end the relationship. 'I feel perfectly normal and happy, then I hear or see something and change into a wild, uncontrollable animal screaming abuse and smashing things. Then I feel terrible – guilty, sorry and embarrassed. It all happens in a flash and I must stop it or my life will be ruined.'

Geoff had learnt his behaviour in childhood from his father who was a belligerent alcoholic. He often beat his wife, smashed furniture and belted Geoff. For years Geoff lived in terror of his father, dreading his return home, drunk and creating havoc. Aged 18 Geoff left home and started life on his own.

His unconscious mind had thousands of buried memories which were triggered by words or actions in the present that mirrored his father's behaviour.

Over a number of sessions we created a concept that 'young Geoff' was living in the unconscious and leapt out when the trigger occurred. Using hypnosis, I guided Geoff into a trance. When he reached the level where the angry 'young Geoff' lived, I talked to 'young Geoff' and discussed how he had learnt his father's anger and how he felt about his father's behaviour. I then talked about Geoff in the present and what was happening in his life and how this was disturbed every time 'young Geoff' 'jumped out'.

We spent many such sessions and over the months Geoff's outbursts became less. His internal conflicts diminished and he became resistant to triggers that previously sparked off outbursts. He continued with

self-hypnosis between sessions and talked to 'young
Geoff' about daily events as well as listening to his
feelings when his father behaved so badly. He praised
'young Geoff' for going through what he did as that
allowed him to be where he is today.

When I last saw him he was much more balanced and
in touch with his feelings and possessed an inner calmness that had previously been foreign to him.

Once you have learnt how to go into a trance it is then time
to decide how to make use of this state for your own needs.
You may choose the trance state to learn more about your
unconscious, alter internal mechanisms or view problems
from a different perspective.

Relaxation

You may choose to go into a trance to relax. This restores
energy and provides a balance for your activities during the
day. Spending 20 minutes feeling really relaxed is refreshing
and re-energising.

Altering self-talk

As we constantly talk to ourselves, generally in a negative
way, the trance state is ideal for improving our internal
language and making it more positive. When you are deeply
relaxed, spend time listening to what you tell yourself. As
you hear negative, critical or judgemental words, change
them to more praising, loving and supportive ones – as if
you were communicating with your best friend.

Use the 20 minutes to talk to yourself in a way that will
help you feel better, more positive, more pleased with

yourself. The aim is to like yourself and appreciate the efforts you are making to deal with life's difficulties. An attitude of 'Well done' for the past and 'You'll do really well' for the future is much more useful than self-criticism.

Talk to different parts of yourself

In trance, as reality is suspended, it is useful to talk to different parts of yourself – either your body or your mind.

Josephine was angry and upset because her hair was falling out. She wore a wig to disguise the areas of baldness and cursed and swore at her head for letting her down, causing her so much shame and humiliation.

I taught her self-hypnosis and after a number of sessions I asked her in a trance to go to her scalp and imagine how it felt. She started to cry saying, 'It feels horrible, it's trying to do its best. It does not want the hair to come out. It is very upset by my criticisms and hatred. It feels very lonely, unloved and isolated.'

When she came out of the trance there was a look of surprise behind her tears. 'I didn't know it felt like that. I didn't realise all my criticisms were causing so much pain. I understand now it is not the fault of my scalp and hair follicles. They are trying their best for me.'

Josephine promised herself she would stop being angry with her scalp, stop using the critical words – both aloud and to herself – and instead develop an attitude of understanding towards her scalp.

Over a period of months her hair loss subsided. It was not perfect but it stabilised. Of all the techniques I used during our consultations, Josephine remarked that this one was the most effective.

Reframing

Often we cannot actually change the situation we are in, but it is possible to improve the way we feel about it by using a technique called 'reframing'. It is one of the most powerful techniques in the psychologists' armoury and is another way of saying 'seeing things from a different point of view'. When you see things from a new perspective they are different and so are you (see Chapter 11).

Louise had a problem with pulling out her eyebrows and eyelashes (in medical terms, trichotillomania). She did this more when she was anxious, but even when she was calm it was a habit that troubled her. She was constantly worried that people would notice and spent a long time using eye make-up to cover the results of her actions.

I taught Louise how to go into a trance and asked her to practise it daily for two weeks. When she returned I asked her to go into a trance once more and when she was deeply relaxed to nod her head.

When she did so I said, 'Louise, you have a problem. You pull out your eyebrows and eyelashes especially when you are nervous. I want us to assess how big the problem really is. I want you to consider your right arm, to think about it and be aware of it. It represents ten per cent of your body and it is very healthy, functions well and works for you. Next I would like you to think of your left arm; another ten per cent works well and is healthy.'

I waited a few minutes while she focused on her healthy arms, before guiding her to her legs, chest, abdomen and back. Again I waited a few minutes for her to focus on these areas.

'Now I want you to focus on your head and neck –

apart from your eyelashes and eyebrows, also working well and healthy.' Another two minutes of silence.

'This leaves 0.001 per cent of your body – 1/1000 that is not working well – your eyelashes and eyebrows. I want you to enjoy the 99.999 per cent of your body that is healthy and working well and not worry about the 0.001 per cent that is not. I would like you to spend some time getting it into perspective and when you have done this come out of the trance.'

After ten minutes in deep thought Louise opened her eyes. 'I've never looked at it like that. It feels much better. I'll work at that every day so I look at things from that perspective.'

I imagine a trance to be similar to a man seeking ways to solve his problem. He rushes everywhere, asks questions, has tests and worries. Just behind him is his unconscious whispering the answer but, as the man is always looking forward, he doesn't hear the soft voice behind. The trance allows him to slow down and find the answer that has been following him all the time.

A 60-year-old businessman sought help from a therapist. He no longer wanted to work every day from nine to five, but he didn't want to retire. The business was running well and he enjoyed it, but he needed some new ideas to keep up with his competitors, and the more time he spent at his desk thinking about this, the more frustrated he became. His hobby was collecting and reading Western magazines. He never seemed to have the time to do this, or when he did have the time he was too tired.

The therapist advised him to work at his business from nine to one, then have lunch. After lunch he was to go back to his office and sit in a comfortable chair on the other side of the room from his desk with a pile of Western magazines and a pencil and paper.

During the afternoon he was to read the Westerns, and to jot down any innovative thoughts about his business that came to his mind. He wasn't to stop and think about them or try to understand what he'd written, but he was to keep reading until four o'clock. At four o'clock he was to look at what he had written and see if the notes were of any use.

The businessman found that he was doing much more for his business in the afternoon while he was reading, than he was doing in the morning when he was trying to think of things that would help. By not consciously try-ing, he was allowing some of the creative knowledge in his unconscious mind to filter through in a most pleasant way.

Coming Out of the Trance

Many people worry that if they go into a trance they may never come out. This fear is not based on any reality.

'What if the hypnotist has a heart attack while I'm in a trance?'

The answer is that you will either return to the normal conscious state or go into a sleep and wake normally. It is useful to have time to come out of a trance so you can adjust to the change just as a diver adjusts to the pressure as he comes up from a dive. Like awakening from a sleep, you need a little while to re-orientate and allow your body and mind to return to daily functions. Some people count slowly from ten back to one, others focus on their in-breaths, while still others imagine coming up from somewhere deep in the mind. It is not really important how you do it as long as you take your time. Once your eyes are open it is a good idea to stretch and rest for a minute or two before getting on with your activities.

If you use self-hypnosis in bed at night it is likely you will move from the trance state into sleep. This is useful if sleep disturbance is a problem, but not if you wish to practise self-hypnosis, as you will be likely to go to sleep instead.

Your creativity is the only limit to the ways you can utilise a trance. The trance state is like the artist's palate: your ability to use the colours will determine the results you achieve. You don't need to be a Picasso to improve things, all you need to do is brighten the picture that is already there.

There is only one world, but there are many ways of looking at it.

4

Words – The Therapist's Tool

Words are loaded pistols.

Jean-Paul Sartre

People who have had problems for months or years and have sought help from tablets, injections and tests without success may well ask, 'How can words help me when all that powerful machinery has failed?'

It's a good question and the answer is difficult to explain. It reminds me of a man who owned a large factory. Something went wrong with the machinery and he had experts in who tested and adjusted it to no avail. He was told about a specialist in these matters who might be of help but who was very expensive.

As the factory was losing money daily the man consulted the specialist who visited the factory, looking here, listening there. Finally, he stopped by one piece of machinery and, taking out a little hammer, tapped it firmly three times. All the machinery began to work perfectly and production was resumed.

When the bill arrived the factory owner was amazed that

it came to £500. He rang the expert to ask why it was so much for just tapping something three times. The answer came back, 'It was £10 for the tapping and £490 for knowing where to tap.'

Perhaps it is the same with hypnosis and words. With modern medical technology and machines like computerised axial tomography (CAT) scanners which cost a million pounds, it seems absurd that words can be more beneficial; especially words that are simpler than the words 'computerised axial tomography scanner'. One would think them ineffectual against a problem or illness that had been going on for a long time.

My own experience is that words are remarkably powerful, and amazing changes will occur with the use of the correct words in a suitable situation. By words I mean either internal dialogue — talking to yourself in your mind (self-talk), or external words spoken by someone else. I could reel off case after case where 'just words' have made the difference between illness and health, but I don't feel that case histories alone would explain it all. So I'll try and analyse how words used in hypnosis can be such a useful method in facilitating change.

Let us consider the mind to be a receiver and converter. Just as a TV set or radio receives waves through the air and converts them to pictures and sounds, the mind receives sounds, pictures, smells and sensations and converts them to thoughts, feelings and actions.

When people are being hypnotised or are practising self-hypnosis, it is the influence of the words, converted to thoughts or feelings, which has such a marked effect. The mind, like a computer, accepts the words in a way that is special for that person. Based on experience, memory and a thousand other factors, the mind will produce a result in the form of a thought, picture or feeling. It could be said that 'word energy' has changed into another form of energy.

The power of this recycled word energy can be seen in many examples. Hitler's oratory had an amazing power over thousands. The words and how they were spoken caused people to behave in a way one wouldn't have thought possible. Go to a religious crusade and note the effect the words have on the listeners.

If someone is dozing in front of the TV and you shout 'fire' in his ear, note how your word energy is changed into anxiety, action and perhaps 'punch on the nose' energy when he realises there is no fire. The word 'fire' has triggered, from previous experience, an alarm reaction. It has mobilised latent energy into activity. This is an absurd example, but it illustrates the power of the word. If we mobilise part of that energy to build self-confidence or to view things from a different angle, then we get a glimpse of the power that words can have on our behaviour.

One consequence of our continuing difficulties is that we use words or thoughts, which may be based on false or outdated assumptions, to cause or maintain our problems. In other words, we hypnotise ourselves into problems with self-talk, so why not use a similar method to hypnotise ourselves out of them.

The words we repeat are like a continuous monologue going on in our minds. Sometimes we are conscious of our self-talk, at other times it drones on beyond our awareness in the depths of the unconscious. If these words are nega-tive, critical, judging or blaming, the outcome will be one of shyness, guilt, anxiety or fear. If the words are caring, loving, supportive and praising, we will feel confident, reassured and positive in our attitudes. So by changing our internal self-talk we can change our attitude and behaviour from negative to positive. This is the power of words and it is used in the process of 'affirmations'. Affirmations are words constructed in a certain way to influence our approach to life positively. The construction has a few simple rules:

1. The affirmation needs to be simple.
2. It needs to be short.
3. It has a rhythm.
4. It involves only positive words.
5. It needs to be in the present tense.

A famous affirmation from a French priest called Emile Coué (1857–1926), who was also a psychologist and pharmacist, runs: 'Every day, in every way, I'm getting better and better.'

This sentence contains positive words, has a rhythm and can be applied to almost any aspect of our life. Coué found that by repeating this sentence many times a day amazing improvements occurred.

You can make your own affirmations to suit your needs. Keep them simple so they can be repeated like a mantra, e.g.:

- I am doing the best I can.
- I learn from each experience.
- I am sensitive, kind and caring.
- Each problem is an opportunity to learn.
- I convert problems into challenges.

The use of suggestions that we repeat to ourselves can facilitate enormous changes in illness. A positive attitude is reflected in the many systems working in the body – it reduces the stress and worry hindering our mind–body connection. All illness, whether psychological or physical, has some involvement of the mind, so making this positive is beneficial to the whole system.

Communication

Communication not only means what we say (the words) but also how we say it – the intonation, rate of speech, body language, power used, loudness or softness, etc.

When we listen to someone talk we hear the words, observe the body language and feel the emotion through the intonation given with the communication. The last part is possibly the most important of the three.

When a therapist is using hypnosis he needs to be aware of all the components of communication and their effects on the patient. If he uses words that trigger fear the patient might return to consciousness to deal with them or put up resistance to further communication.

A woman who was feeling depressed decided to turn to hypnotherapy for help. The therapist was very direct and after 20 minutes told her that her problems were due to the fact she did not have children. He then advised her and her husband to start a family straightaway and her depression would be cured. She left the appointment feeling annoyed and confused that she had received such a recommendation after only the first session.

No wonder she was upset. In this example, it is clear that the therapist had not had time to understand the factors involved in the woman's life and his advice had been bewildering rather than reassuring as intended.

The Power of Words

Imagine the body and mind are like a radio. The radio normally broadcasts music and programmes which can be heard satisfactorily and which provide entertainment. One day the radio sounds terrible, the voices are blurred, the sound is poor and the music is grating. Perhaps the set needs a new valve or spare part, perhaps a technician is required to correct the fault, or perhaps just a slight adjustment of the tuning and volume may rectify the problem. If the radio is not properly tuned we don't take it to the shop for an expensive overhaul, we only do that if all the minor adjustments fail to produce the desired effect.

So it is with hypnosis, where the words spoken by the therapist or by yourself may provide the 'fine tuning' necessary to overcome the difficulty. The words used by great orators and preachers rely on the powerful blasting of speeches heavily laden with emotion to create their effect. This is not necessary in hypnosis where the quietly spoken word (like the man tapping in the right place), the relaxing story or peaceful sounds may provide the basis for the mind to work out an alternative view of the situation.

How is it done? The elements are simple but it is not a simple process. The question of how hypnosis works has been discussed for centuries and no real agreement has been reached. Many theories shed some light on the matter and each has a grain of truth, but none explains it satisfactorily. I will try and clarify a few aspects involved in the mechanism of hypnosis, to show how benefits may be obtained. Let's look at an arbitrary situation and study the components to discover where and how hypnosis may be of use.

John and Sue have been going steady for six months. He is nervous and shy but the relationship is going well and he is very happy to have someone like Sue to be his constant companion. One night he drinks too much and fails at making love. He starts to worry, he's 28 – perhaps he is too old, perhaps it will happen again. What will she think? She may leave me – and so on. Next time he tries, the worry and negative self-talk ensure that he fails again and so completes his internal self-fulfilling prophecy.

He cautiously talks to a few of his friends who try to reassure him, but he doesn't believe their comments and things go from bad to worse. The worry spreads through the relationship, affecting many other aspects of it.

John's 'self-talk' is convincing him he is impotent and is maintaining that conviction. The 'self-talk' is on an unconscious level so reassurance from his friends will not reach it. Hypnosis allows a message to sink to a deeper level in the mind. The fact that the positive self-talk in a hypnotic trance reaches the unconscious, means it can override the negative tape repeating, 'I'm no good, I'll fail again', and replace it with, 'I'm normal and healthy.'

The words used in hypnosis bypass conscious resistance, so John's negative attitude need not be dealt with on a conscious level. Talking to him while he is relaxed means that the general anxiety and tension surrounding this very sensitive subject will be less. Explaining to his unconscious mind that he performed well previously, and will be able to do so again, is very reassuring and builds confidence. Encouraging him not to try to perform will enable him to act more naturally. Permitting the problem to assume a suitable perspective in his life will allow him to regain his confidence and overcome his difficulty.

This situation arises in many of the adversities we encounter. The 'common-sense' attitude delivered on a conscious level – 'pull your socks up and get on with it' – generally has either a minimal or negative effect by adding guilt to an already fragile situation.

One view as to how hypnosis can be effective may be its use in overcoming conscious resistance. As we grow, through years of painstaking trial and error, to achieve the position we are now in, we don't take kindly to advice from outsiders who tell us to behave differently. This resistance to change is something we may not be aware of. According to our belief system we will have sound logical reasons for refuting any advice offered. For a multitude of reasons – fear, lack of confidence, disbelief or plain stubbornness – we cling to our position as a mountaineer clings to the rockface if he is unsure of his footing.

So it is with patients and their predicaments. They cling to their situation, resisting advice either from themselves or from others.

Suzie, aged 25, has had asthma, for which she uses an inhaler, since the age of four. She also has eczema and uses cream to minimise the problem. She knows her condition gets worse when she is tense or upset, and has been told by many people to relax. She has tried various methods of relaxation, but gets frightened at being on her own and is constantly on the go.

The advice she has been given seems sound enough, but something in Suzie prevents her from following it. This could be termed a 'resistance' to trying something beneficial due to an unknown fear.

When I saw her, we came to an agreement that she would spend ten minutes a day for two weeks doing self-hypnosis, and then we would review the situation. During her self-hypnosis she discovered a number of things about her childhood. Two important things were: first, that something unpleasant happened to her when she was on her own at about the time the eczema started at the age of four; and second, on another occasion she became very angry with someone and lost control.

Discussing these two events and trying to fit them into the picture, Suzie believed her fear of being alone related to the early incident. When she was ten she had made a commitment to herself that, because she had once lost control, she would never be angry or lose her temper again.

So her resistance to change was due to two internal directions: do not be on your own or something terrible may happen as it did when you were four; and do not express your anger or you may lose control as you did when you were ten.

After some discussion she agreed to spend time by herself either doing self-hypnosis or relaxing, and also to explore gradually how she could express her feelings.

In this way she could circumvent resistance and, using positive 'self-talk', direct herself with the following: 'Now I am 25 it is OK to be alone from time to time' and 'Expressing feelings, such as anger, is allowable at 25 as I could make sure I do not lose control.'

The eczema and asthma were the result of her inability to create an outlet for normal feelings and experiences. As she learnt to unblock her resistance to change, the eczema and asthma steadily improved. The positive words she fed into her internal dialogue allowed her skin to clear gradually and the spasms in her chest to subside.

It is not only in hypnosis that we can observe the remarkable effect words have on our behaviour. I was playing tennis against an old friend. He was serving really well and I had great difficulty returning his serves. He was four games ahead in the first set and as we changed ends I said, 'You are really serving well, how do you do it?'

He then served double fault after double fault and his game collapsed. His mind was trying to analyse 'how he did it' and so his rhythm and serving pattern became stiff and unnatural.

My remark was indeed innocent but after the game he commented, 'You bloody hypnotists, why don't you keep your remarks to the consulting rooms!'

The Effect of Our Early Life

Past experiences that remain in the unconscious may influence our present. These memories may be outside conscious awareness and retrieved only during a hypnosis session. There is generally an intense emotional component from the past playing a role in the present problem.

Julia is a 40-year-old housewife with four children ranging from 6 to 16. Her life has the usual ups and downs and she deals with these very well. She is bright and cheerful and appears thoughtful and concerned, but she has been troubled for years with migraine headaches every one or two weeks. These are so severe that she needs to lie down in a darkened room for most of the day. Over the years she has had tests and treatment. She was taking tablets which did ease the pain but had side-effects that she did not like. She was also becoming more and more frustrated by her dependence on drugs.

There did not seem anything obvious in her present situation which was causing the headaches. Her relationship with her husband and children was good and she did not seem to be using self-talk to precipitate the migraine.

She was a good and willing subject for hypnosis and agreed to learn self-hypnosis. She described the migraines as 'punishing headaches', which keep me in bed for the day'. The word 'punishing' seemed to have some significance, so I was not surprised when she returned after two weeks of practising self-hypnosis to tell me that she believed the migraine was due to something she had done when she was young.

In a trance, she went back to when she was eight years old. She remembered playing in the park, being swung around by the park attendant. He had his hand under her dress but she said this was only to hold her properly whilst swinging her around. Her mother reacted angrily when Julia told her about it and went to the police to complain. The man was brought to court and little Julia had to identify him and say what happened. Even though she wailed through her tears that he'd done nothing wrong, he was sacked from his job. She remembered the very sad look he gave her as he was led from the courtroom, and the extreme guilt she had felt at having caused so much trouble was still with her. Her face filled with grief and tears ran down her face as she told her story in the trance.

I let her cry for a few minutes and then gently suggested that perhaps it was not all her fault; perhaps she behaved as a normal child would have behaved, but her parents' fears took things out of her hands. Even if she was guilty, did she need to be punished with migraine after all these years? She spent some time altering the message on her internal tape recorder and helping the young Julia in her mind understand that there was no need to be punished any more.

Why it took so long for the punishment to occur I do not know. Perhaps it was a particularly happy time in her life and hence the 'computer judge' decided to carry out the sentence passed years before. Learning about this was of great benefit to Julia who gradually, over some months, let go of her unnecessary guilt from the past and her migraines subsided.

Imprinting

The words which are the vehicle for these situations often evolve from simple circumstances. At other times more complex scenes have occurred for the literature of the mind to be set in concrete. One example of the power of words is a situation called imprinting. This is related to the imprinting that occurs in birds and animals which has been brilliantly studied by the Austrian zoologist Konrad Lorenz (1903–89) and others.

Imprinting is a term used to describe the powerful way words are planted in the back of the mind and their effect remains there for years, sometimes even for a lifetime. An imprint is:

1. A command made by
2. someone in authority
3. to someone under stress or very frightened.

Such a command or imprint may go deeply into the mind, leaving its mark there long after the initial situation has been forgotten. The command continues to exert its authority for years as a form of compulsion, being followed without question.

Here is an example of the effect words can have in the form of an imprint on someone very nervous someone in authority.

Mrs Jacobs was in hospital having a baby. I was looking after her and delivered a normal baby girl. The baby developed a problem with her chest and was put in an incubator to help her breathing.

Mrs Jacobs was understandably anxious about her baby and developed nervous diarrhoea, going to the toilet many times during the night. There was a very officious Sister on duty who aggressively blamed her for disturbing the other patients.

Mrs Jacobs became more anxious and the diarrhoea persisted. After a few days I decided to let her go home to see if it would settle down. By this time the baby was well. The night before her discharge, the aggressive Sister came to her and said, 'If you go home tomorrow, you'll be sick for a very long time.'

She was! For months and months she had abdominal pains that defied any diagnosis, in spite of all the investigations performed. Specialists prodded and probed, looked into every orifice, X-rayed her from top to toe, and took pieces of her bowel to examine. No abnormality could be found.

The imprint of the Sister had taken effect and there seemed nothing we could do about it. In hypnosis it was revealed that the Sister's words were still having a powerful effect and they seemed to be locked into her mind. I could not help her change them.

I last saw Mrs Jacobs a year after her baby was born. She continued to have tests and treatment for her abdominal pains and I was still receiving letters from specialists trying to find the cause of this distressed woman's problems.

Often this imprinting happens in childhood and is lost in the backwoods of the mind. It may be reinforced by other words or events and the time between the command and the carrying out of the command may be many years.

I saw an overweight woman of 30 who had struggled since she was very small to lose the fat which continued to be a burden to her. She had tried every diet and every club related to weight loss and had consulted numerous helpers in the field of obesity.

During a session with self-hypnosis she went back to the time when she was four years old. She was fat at this time and her mother dragged her along to a doctor for help. The doctor was overpowering and very frightening to the little girl, who was terrified by the sights and smells of his surgery. After examining the girl, the doctor said to her mother, 'She's just a fat girl and will be fat for the rest of her life.' This edict somehow registered with the child as a prophecy which must come true. It had the three components of an imprint: a figure of authority, a frightened child and a command.

The unconscious takes words very literally. The doctor said she would be fat for the rest of her life, that is, *if she got thin she would die*. So she started on a see-saw battle, her conscious mind struggling to lose weight, her unconscious terrified of losing weight and dying. The battle continued in a similar way on many fronts, keeping the imprinted command in mind at all times. A loss of weight would be rapidly followed by a binge.

There needs to be 'fallow ground' for these imprints to take hold. We have all been given commands by authoritarian figures whilst being nervous and they have not controlled our lives. The fertile soil of low self-esteem, guilt and perhaps a basic inherent belief in the edict even before it is spoken, may be necessary.

Often these imprints may be altered by repeated self-hypnosis and by 'updating' the unconscious mind, reassuring it about the fears it has harboured for years. At other times the imprint seems to persist in spite of the various manoeuvres available to patient and therapist. The fear of changing may be too great to allow any light to be shed on the powerful command from the past.

Language From a Deeper Level

The words we use may well indicate what is going on at different levels of the mind. Slips of the tongue tell us unconscious beliefs and reasoning. Words that seem a little out of context may be the way the unconscious is trying to communicate with the listener.

Mildred was referred to me by her GP for fears and anxiety. The day before her appointment her sister rang to tell me she believed Mildred was interfered with by her father when she was young. She said Mildred might deny this but the general view of the family was that it had definitely happened. When Mildred arrived I mentioned her sister had rung (I always tell patients if someone has contacted me).

'Oh. I suppose she went on about that episode with Dad when I was young,' she remarked, 'but that's all poppycock.' Now poppycock is not a word I regularly hear so I paid attention to it. Was the unconscious telling me her sister's story was true? I kept that in mind as I treated Mildred and over a period of time and a number of hypnotic sessions it became obvious that she had indeed been interfered with by her father.

Altering Self-talk

Once you have established what self-talk the unconscious is using, you can then try to alter it through hypnosis to provide new thoughts that are relevant for your current situation.

Daphne was 50 and had little confidence. She rushed around a lot and constantly used phrases like 'I have to', 'I must', 'I ought to', etc.

We discussed this fact and how it was influencing her life. I asked her to close her eyes and imagine who was in her head telling her she 'must', 'should' or 'ought to'. She sat quietly for a minute then smiled and said, 'I can see a sharp-looking and angular woman with a threatening finger pointing at me telling me what to do.'

'Ask her what her name is.'

Daphne smiles again, 'She says she is called Harriet. What a strange name, I don't know anyone called Harriet.'

'Ask Harriet how old you were when she became part of you.'

'I was little, very little, about five.'

'And why did Harriet become part of you, when you were five?'

'To make me do my work at school. I think I was lazy so Harriet was necessary.'

'Ask Harriet how old she thinks you are now'

'She says I'm eight, but I know I'm 50.'

'She doesn't know that. Help her to know you are now grown up and don't need her to tell you what to do.'

'She is really surprised that I'm as old as I am and she is shrinking as I talk to her.'

'Would it be possible to have a part inside who praises rather than criticises?'

'Yes that would be much better.'

'Who would you like to have in there as a praiser?'

'Josie, a friend of mine, is always saying nice things about people. I'd love her to be in my head talking to me.'

'Good. Imagine Josie inside your head taking over Harriet's role.'

'Yes, she is there and Harriet has shrunk right down and is sitting in the corner.'

'Good, I'd like you to spend some time each day making sure Josie is with you talking to you and that Harriet remains shrunk and in the corner.'

After the session Daphne used 'should', 'have to' and 'must' less frequently. She felt better about herself and her self-confidence grew week by week.

It was the controlling words that led me on the trail to discovering Harriet and enabling Daphne to alter her self-talk from one of criticism to one of praise.

The fact that words have such a powerful influence on the way we feel explains why the hypnotherapist uses them as a powerful tool for change.

Using a trance to allow conversations with the unconscious means that the mechanism for change can go right to the heart of the matter, implementing new thoughts and feelings more appropriate for life in the present.

5

Self-hypnosis

The mind is a gold mine of inexhaustible abilities. The fortune of the fortunate is knowing how to find them.

Brian Roet

If you give a man a fish you give him a meal. If you teach him how to fish you give him a livelihood.

Proverb

All hypnosis is self-hypnosis. By learning how to go into a trance you gain access to the many treasures the mind possesses. I liken it to brushing your teeth; you go to the dentist to fix any problems then brush your teeth daily to prevent any more occurring.

One of the major benefits of self-hypnosis is that you make quiet time for yourself on a daily basis. Notice I use the word 'make' not 'find'. It is a lot easier to have a commitment to make 20 minutes a day for yourself than it is to find it. For example, 'I must do some self-hypnosis, but I've got so many other things I have to do first.' The day goes by and as you drag yourself to bed tired and exhausted from the daily activities you say, 'Oh. I didn't get round to doing that self-hypnosis, I'm too tired now, I'll do it tomorrow.' Like the good intentions of dieting, the mantra is 'I'll start tomorrow.'

As I was saying, the 'quiet time' aspect of self-hypnosis is a major benefit. It means you are moving from the 'trying state' of mind to the 'being state'. In anatomical terms you are moving from left brain to right brain.

The benefits of self-hypnosis are many. You can use the relaxation component, the quiet 'being' component to balance your busy life. You can use the trance state to promote positive self-talk in the form of affirmations. You can connect with the unconscious to review the previous 24 hours. You can set a pattern for the next 24 hours, programming your mind to be positive and successful. You can focus on your feelings and view them from the perspective of solitude and calmness. Self-hypnosis can help you:

- To sleep better use self-hypnosis once you are in bed or play a sleep tape as you turn out the light. Use positive suggestions of relaxing, sleeping until the morning, and waking refreshed and in a positive frame of mind.

- Using time which is normally wasted in travel to and from work as a passenger in a train or bus (not as the driver of a car). Sitting in a trance during a train journey is a great way of reclaiming wasted time. Programme yourself for the day ahead, looking at solutions for specific problems you may encounter.

- Before a normally tense-making experience, which may range from business meetings to meeting new people. Many professional sportsmen and performers use self-hypnosis to create positive attitudes before an event. A dress rehearsal in the mind boosts confidence.

- In the bath at night to review the day's activities, observe positive aspects of the day and put into perspective any negative occurrences – as if you are writing a confidence-building mental diary.

- To look at future experiences in a positive, relaxing way. During pregnancy to anticipate an easy, joyful delivery of a healthy baby. Before an exam or a driving test to imagine a calm, successful performance with a positive outcome.

The following 20 steps are involved in using self-hypnosis. Remember the most important part is *making time* on a daily basis.

1. Ascertain what you wish to achieve in the allotted time. It may be to relax, remove tension or for a more specific complaint such as to relieve a headache. Be concise, realistic and specific in your aims. Approaching self-hypnosis as a cure-all or a happiness-maker will be met with failure.

2. Choose an appropriate time and place. It may be helpful to set a routine for the same time and place each day. It should be somewhere where you feel secure and will not be disturbed. It may be your bedroom, the train, the toilet at work, the bath, the car in the car park.

3. Make sure those around you will not interfere with your session. Do not approach it with the attitude, 'I've got to spend this ten minutes relaxing but I'll be late for work and I've got so many other things to do.'

4. Ten to 20 minutes a day is an average time spent on self-hypnosis and many people set their alarms to 'reclaim' 20 minutes of sleep for this activity.

5. Do not do it when you are exhausted and nearly asleep as the relaxing aspect will send you to sleep. Sleep and self-hypnosis are not the same thing.

6. Choose a position that is comfortable – lying on the floor or sitting in an armchair with your head supported. If you find you are going to sleep choose a less comfortable position next time.

7. Focus your eyes on a point on the ceiling (it is preferable if your eyes are looking upwards), and stay staring at that point for a minute or two until your eyelids become tired.

8. When you are ready let your eyelids close and focus your attention on your breathing. As you breathe out allow a feeling of drifting/floating to permeate your body. Make your focus internal so any external noise can waft away.

9. Allow whatever happens to happen – thoughts, feelings, self-talk. Do not try to analyse or make logical sense of them, do not try and stop them; move into a *being* state.

10. Have in your mind your problem or what you wish to accomplish by the self-hypnosis session. Talk to yourself about this before you go into a trance, then let it float around undirected. Do not try and achieve any result consciously; trying is the opposite of self-hypnosis.

11. As you drift into the altered state be a passive observer of any thoughts or feelings you have. They may not be related to your current problem: do not worry – the picture will become clearer with time, piece by piece, just as a jigsaw puzzle does. Direct your mind inward rather than outward.

12. Enjoy the relaxing feeling that goes with self-hypnosis and appreciate the benefit of the 'oasis in the desert of stress' for a few minutes. Perhaps you may recognise some components of your problem in the

dream language of the unconscious, but these may come to you later on during the day or night.

13. Remain in that state for 10 to 20 minutes (or however long is suitable) as a receiver of messages or no message at all. Allow a feeling of parallel awareness to be present. Do not expect too much – many things may be occurring beyond your conscious recognition.

14. You may talk to yourself in a positive way, praising, promoting, reassuring, as if talking to a shy child, in order to remove guilt, fear or negative attitudes. Look at things from different angles and find an avenue to establish confidence and success.

15. Do not hope for great changes after each session. A small change in attitude each day will bring about improvement in time. Constant dripping wears away the stone. Continually assessing and worrying that there is no progress will ensure that there will be none.

16. When you are ready, come out of the trance in any way suitable. By counting slowly from ten back to one is a good way to start; in time you will find this may be unnecessary.

17. Do not let your conscious mind dissect and analyse different aspects of the trance. This is very important. Enjoy whatever feeling you have for a minute or two before getting on with your daily routine.

18. If you are a deep subject and feel disorientated when coming out of a trance, give yourself a few minutes to return to normal before getting up and carrying on with things.

19. In time you may find yourself drifting in and out of a trance for a few seconds during the day when appropriate. Your experiences and abilities to use self-hypnosis will vary from time to time, depending on the situations arising in your life.

20. As it becomes part of your routine you may not need self-hypnosis on a daily basis but rather wait for a specific problem to occur before using the combined conscious–unconscious approach of a trance to deal with it.

To hypnotise oneself to go into a trance is an individual experience. It may be compared to a surfer setting out to catch a wave. The novice surfer wades into the sea, swimming out to where the 'big ones' are. He swims out ten metres and is buffeted back by an incoming wave. He tries again and struggles out a few more metres before being washed shorewards by the next wave. This process continues as he slowly makes his way out, becoming more and more exhausted with each stroke. When he eventually reaches a place where he can catch a wave in, he is so tired he hasn't the energy to enjoy it.

As he learns, he realises that swimming out to catch a wave may be easier. Every time a wave comes towards him he takes in a deep breath and dives below the surface; it is calm there and the powerful force of the wave passes ineffectually over him. He bobs up again two seconds later to continue his outward journey.

Time and time again he allows the incoming breakers to flow over him as he gradually swims further out. He floats on the swell waiting for the right wave to take him in. As it arrives he turns shorewards, swims powerfully for a few strokes, so his momentum is the same as the wave's, then relaxes and enjoys the exhilarating ride to the shore, using the energy of the wave to carry him effortlessly there.

Self-hypnosis is like the surfer ducking under the wave. It enables us to conserve energy and the 'big waves' of life to pass by. By going into a trance state regularly we can avoid much of the tension continually swirling around us. We can let it pass by while we catch our breath for the next 'wave' of the day.

Therapeutic Components of Self-hypnosis

Relaxation

As many of our problems are the result of stress and tension, utilising the relaxation component of self-hypnosis is of great benefit. By going into a trance we automatically lessen the nervous impulses travelling around our body, causing the muscles to relax. This component can be enhanced by 'talking' to different parts of the body and guiding them to relax: 'My arm is relaxed and comfortable' or 'My head feels calm and tranquil'.

These messages act as a signal for the mind to decrease the tension in the body just as calming music or a warm bath does. The relaxation component is very important and is incorporated with other techniques in order to maximise the benefits. For example, it can lessen pre-menstrual tension. Often just the relaxation on its own is enough to restore the balance in a stressed and anxious person.

Improving self-talk

We are constantly talking to ourselves about things we do, imagine and feel. This self-talk is often negative and pessimistic. Self-hypnosis is a very good vehicle for implanting positive words into the deeper layers of the mind. If these words are in the form of brief sentences they are called affirmations (see p. 41). Like poetry the wording is received on a deeper, more emotional level and can be more effective than if spoken on a conscious level.

Julie was a pretty 30-year-old woman whose mother had been depressed and lonely since her husband left when Julie was ten years old. She came to see me for help in becoming more confident. She struggled whenever there was conflict or confrontation and had developed a 'victim' personality, believing she had no control over her life, was always a loser and could never say 'no' to any request.

We spent a number of sessions looking at her past and present life and her aims. A constant refrain that appeared was the message, 'I'm no good, I don't have a right to voice an opinion.'

She learnt self-hypnosis initially to lessen the tension and anxiety that were her constant companions. The relaxation component eased the pain and she looked forward to the 'oasis of calm' when she came home from work. Her technique was to give herself a treat by having a long and luxurious bath using scented oils and lighted candles. Whilst soaking in the hot water she would relax completely and reflect on any positive events from the day.

We then looked at her self-talk and started to eliminate all the negative components. She gradually created her own phrases which suited her aims. She built up a series of affirmations which replaced the negative self-talk she had learnt from her mother. She removed the 'should nots' and 'must nots' from her vocabulary and replaced them with, 'I'm as good as anyone else', 'It really doesn't matter if I make mistakes as I will learn from them', 'I will treat myself as I treat my best friend', 'When I say "no" to others I'm saying "yes" to myself and I'm the most important person to myself'.

It took many months of self-hypnosis with lots of ups and downs but eventually Julie started to like herself and respect the views she held. She took some risks and found that the world did not collapse. She realised that improving her self-talk made a great difference to the way she felt.

Visualisation

As well as talking to ourselves we also have a projectionist in the back of our mind showing us pictures of the past, present and future. Sometimes these projectionists have a very negative slant on life and show us pictures that are restrictive, frightening or that produce guilt or anger. We may see failure, embarrassment or criticism occurring in the future and so avoid doing things. We may see blame or failure and so become depressed. We may see rejection and have low self-esteem.

It is possible to alter these pictures, change the projectionist and create pictures that are more appropriate, positive and helpful. This technique is called visualisation which is just another word for imagination, and the trance state is a very good vehicle for improving our internal video library. Often this library is formed from previous experiences and plays a major role in how we deal with future experiences.

If someone has had a very bumpy, frightening aeroplane flight it is possible that when a future journey is planned the internal projectionist, although aiming to protect us, will show terrifying pictures of that previous flight. This generates such fear that it is difficult to contemplate boarding the plane.

A childhood experience with a dog may cause the projectionist to show pictures of large, frightening dogs that induce a phobia about them.

Using self-hypnosis we can change the pictures so they are more helpful and appropriate to our life in the present. We are not denying that the previous experience occurred but what we are doing is saying, 'Yes, that did happen, but I was young then and I've developed more strengths and can cope better. Just because one dog frightened me it doesn't mean every dog needs to be frightening.'

And so we use our imagination in the trance to see dogs or plane flights from a positive, optimistic perspective. We replace the out-of-date pictures with ones that are more suitable and helpful.

Dissociation

In a trance many people describe 'being there' and 'being somewhere else' at the same time. This is called 'parallel awareness' or 'dissociation'. 'I knew I was here in this room and I was also lying on a beach in Spain.'

This ability to dissociate is an important factor in self-hypnosis and varies from person to person. To let go, to suspend critical judgement, to use imagination and allow the benefits of self-hypnosis to be explored, all play a part in the hypnotic trance.

A good example of this parallel awareness arose when I saw Les, a 50-year-old builder who was suffering from panic attacks and anxiety. I asked him what his favourite hobby was and I was pleased when he said fly-fishing as that is my favourite hobby too. I said I was going to teach him to go into a trance and he could practise self-hypnosis daily at home.

I asked him to close his eyes and in time I started telling him he was beside a lovely mountain stream casting his line out into the sparkling water. I described the sounds of the birds, the feel of the breeze and the river splashing over rocks. I talked for a little while and then suggested he lay down on a grassy bank by the river and go into a deeply relaxed state. I then talked about ways he could deal with the stress in his life in a calm and relaxed manner. When he came out of the trance I asked him how he enjoyed it.

'It was fantastic,' he replied, 'I was near this beautiful mountain stream casting my line out and I hooked a really big trout. I was reeling him in but some idiot kept telling me to lie down on the grass. I kept resisting him until I'd landed a massive 3lb brown trout, then I lay down and relaxed as I'd been directed.'

Les's story is a good example of parallel awareness – he was able to fish and accept a strange voice telling him to lie down without realising how ludicrous this actually was. His critical, analytical mind had gone off duty and he was accepting my suggestions (or resisting them when I said to lie down) without logical examination.

Stage-hypnotists make use of this phenomenon when subjects act in a humorous way which is contrary to their personality. People who are normally shy suspend that aspect and order people around. In medical hypnosis this facility can be put to use to overcome hurdles that are otherwise difficult to surmount. One way of using this dissociation is, in a trance, to imagine that someone else 'over there' is going through the difficulty while you are watching from 'here'. All the emotional conflicts affect 'him over there' and you can be an observer of the procedure without suffering the painful feelings involved.

I used that technique with a very nervous man who had been trying for months to pluck up the courage to ask his boss for a rise. He was a good hypnotic subject and I taught him self-hypnosis. Every day he practised imagining he was watching 'the other him' going through the motions (and emotions) of asking his boss for a rise. This 'other him' felt all the nervous tension involved while my patient sat and watched as an unemotional observer.

On the big day, when he had an appointment to see his boss, he remained in a trance throughout the whole procedure. He got his rise and when he saw me later on he said his only problem was not smiling during the interview.

'For some reason,' he said, 'it reminded me of a Laurel and Hardy-type film, where the nervous employee asks the stern boss for a rise. All the time I was in his office I imagined him as the character in the film and me as the 'fall guy', all of which I found very funny. At one stage I had to cough to avoid laughing.'

He had used the dissociation technique not only in the practice sessions but in the actual event itself. I received a note from him some months later saying he had found many opportunities for using this technique of 'distancing' himself from his problems.

Imagine that when you were born a small candle was placed in your vital centre (which is wherever you imagine that place to be). This is a special candle, a little like the Olympic eternal flame. It will not be extinguished until you die. However, its brightness, radiant light and warmth are dependent upon being tended properly. It needs care, attention and respect in order to grow as you grow. If it remains as that tiny initial candle its effect will be lost as the body grows. What would be sufficient for a baby is inadequate for an adult. Many things could happen which would dampen the flame, reduce its intensity and threaten to blow it out. Just like a candle in the breeze, it flickers and wavers constantly. If it receives inadequate attention in the form of time, praise, acceptance or respect, it will become stunted and drop behind the growth rate of other parts. Less candle-power may be a way of describing our lack of self-confidence.

Self-hypnosis could be regarded as directly tending that candle in an appropriate way, giving it the time, oxygen and protection that will allow it to stabilise, grow and become powerful enough to resist the winds of fate which continually blow.

During self-hypnosis one may concentrate on that 'essential candle', allowing the feeling of warmth and exuberance to grow and last long after the trance. This candle-power will not only be felt by you but others will notice the improvement, the 'radiance' coming from that internal source of energy, the different attitude not only of you to others but of them to you.

Tony was shy, lacked confidence and was continually putting himself down. He did not like himself and his underlying anger radiated wherever he went. People kept their distance and he had acquaintances rather than friends.

When I asked him how he had learnt to dislike himself so much, he said, 'My Dad was a lot like me. He was always critical of Mum and me. We could never do anything right.'

'Could you give me an example?' I asked.

Tony thought for a while and then said, 'Yes. I remember when I was 12. I was very keen on swimming and practised very hard for the school sports. On sports day I swam with all my might and won my race. I was so excited. I ran over to Dad and said, "Did you see that, Dad, I won?"

'"Yes Tony," he replied, "I saw that, but do you realise it is the best swimmers who drown?"

'I was devastated. All I wanted was some praise for all my effort and then he said that. Did he want me to be a bad swimmer so I wouldn't drown?'

We discussed Dad and his influence and how Tony had been negatively brainwashed by him. I asked Tony to do self-hypnosis daily to reprogramme his mind in a positive way. In a trance he was to repeat that he was normal and healthy. His attitudes and behaviour were fine and any negative input his mind was storing from his father would be diminished.

I asked him to visualise his 'essential candle' deep within and give it the nurturing it had been deprived of in childhood. He was to help it become stronger and larger and brighter.

Tony did as I asked and we continued to have sessions discussing and reducing the role his negative father had played in his early life. He kept the memory of the swimming race as a yardstick of the influence he had received.

With time Tony's attitude to life changed. He did indeed nourish the internal candle so that he felt much better about himself and the world around him.

I cannot urge you too strongly to develop a routine where you spend 20 minutes a day quietly reflecting, being passive and relaxing so that you give yourself the balance necessary to realise your true potential.

6

Deep Trance Phenomena

Reality testing is the feedback of our senses responding to the world around us. This is diminished in hypnosis allowing the unconscious to enter our mind's arena.

Brian Roet

When a patient enters a deep trance they experience a variety of sensations called 'deep trance phenomena'. The art of the therapist is to use whatever happens in trance to help the patient gain insight, strength or resources which they can apply to the symptom troubling them.

A young woman was unhappy in her job, but every move she made to leave was negated by guilt and so she stayed.

In a trance she felt dizzy and uncomfortable and I said to her, 'Do you think your unconscious is trying to tell you something?'

'What do you mean?' she replied.

'Stay focused on the dizziness and learn what it is trying to tell you.'

After a while she opened her eyes.

'That was most unpleasant, the words "Going around in circles" came into my mind. What does that mean?'

'What do you think it may mean in relation to your job?'

'I suppose I'm going around in circles trying to leave my job. That feels right.'

We then discussed ways of 'not going around in circles' and she made some decisions and commitments that helped her leave.

People respond much better to lessons they learn from their own experiences than from being told what to do, and in the case above the patient's conscious mind could not argue with the fact she felt she was going around in circles, because that feeling was real in the trance.

The phenomena occurring in a deep trance are:

Relaxation

Patients may feel so relaxed they are unable to move. Their arms and legs become very heavy, their eyelids feel so relaxed they cannot open their eyes. Some people feel so restful they go to sleep. This feeling is extremely pleasant and is in direct contrast to the anxiety generally associated with their symptoms. Many patients seek help just to gain this deep relaxation as it provides an oasis during the day when practised regularly as self-hypnosis.

Age Regression

People can be taken back in time in two separate ways, either to 'relive' an experience as if it is actually happening in the present, or remember it in a vivid way whilst being aware it is a memory.

If the experience is 'relived' the speech pattern and mannerisms are that of the child concerned. If a different language was spoken in childhood, the patient may revert to this language (much to the consternation of the therapist!).

If it is a 'vivid memory' the details are very clear, the experience being seen from a different perspective. During regression patients often become aware of abilities previously unrecognised, as they have been lying dormant and inaccessible to the conscious mind. Following this recognition, they can be incorporated into attitudes and behaviour in any situation that may arise.

Age Progression

This means taking the trance subject into the future to view his life from this perspective. Present-day aims and activities can be taken to a positive outcome and stepping stones to the future envisaged.

A technique I commonly use when people are in conflict about their behaviour is to put them in a trance and ask them to imagine two different roads into the future. They progress along one, then the other, to discover how they feel when alternative attitudes are experienced.

If a person comes to see me to stop smoking, I hypnotise them and ask them to imagine how it would be for their lungs if they continue smoking 20 cigarettes a day for the next ten years. I then ask them to be aware how their lungs would feel if they stopped smoking and breathed normal air for the next ten years. This age progression helps their resolve to stop smoking.

Analgesia

It is possible to make a part of the body numb during hypnosis. In this way operations can be performed without an anaesthetic.

Pain clinics sometimes have hypnotherapists in their team, as the mind is a very powerful force in relieving pain. Many people are able to reduce their medication when practising self-hypnosis on a regular basis (see Chapter 14).

Dissociation

Dissociation (see p. 66) means the separating of conscious and unconscious minds as occurs when we are driving. Our thoughts drift on to various subjects whilst our unconscious does the driving.

This phenomenon is an integral part of hypnosis and can be used by the therapist in a variety of ways. The unconscious can speak, lift an arm, feel feelings and remember things whilst the conscious is thinking about something completely different and may be unaware of the actions of the unconscious.

Arm levitation is frequently used to demonstrate disso-ciation. On a suggestion the arm rises of its own accord, completely out of control of the conscious mind which becomes an observer of the rising arm. The patient can have his eyes open and generally a smile of disbelief crosses his face, as if he is unable to believe what is happening.

Catalepsy

When we focus intensely on something we often 'forget to move' and remain motionless. As hypnosis is a state of internal focusing, people in a trance become motionless – normal movement, fidgeting, sighing, swallowing, looking around, all cease. They develop a fixed gaze and regular breathing and if an arm is lifted by the therapist it will remain in that position. This is called catalepsy and indicates the person is in a deep trance.

This state can be used by the therapist to help the patient see how 'stuck' they are in their problem, and how they can develop ways and means of overcoming this impasse.

Amnesia

The ability to forget things is part of the mind's way of dealing with information. It would be impossible to remember consciously everything we have ever experienced, so the mind uses amnesia to let go of the majority of our experiences.

In hypnosis it is possible to direct patients to forget things, and in the process help them realise on a deeper level that they are able to forget traumatic memories that are causing problems.

Time Distortion

Most people believe the trance experience is shorter than it actually is. This is called time distortion; often a trance lasting 30 minutes feels like five. The clock in the mind, unlike the one on the wall, is able to vary time depending on the situation.

> *Time is*
> *Too slow for those who wait.*
> *Too swift for those who fear.*
> *Too long for those who grieve.*
> *Too short for those who rejoice.*

And so it is in a trance; the variability of time can be utilised to minimise the time painful experiences are re-experienced, to lengthen the time joyful memories are recalled, to reduce the time till resolution occurs.

Often a 'time line' may be used as a technique in trance. In this process the patient is asked to imagine a line from birth to death, and to focus on his problem in the present on that line. The therapist can then guide the patient to realise the time factors involved in many of his problems and put them into a perspective related to the rest of his life.

Hallucination

Situations are often imagined clearly and distinctly in a trance 'as if they are real'. We can create positive hallucinations where we experience something that is not there. We can do this through any of the senses – taste, sight, smell, sound, touch. We can also have negative hallucinations where we do not experience something that is actually present.

I often use this phenomenon with people who have low self-confidence. In a trance I ask them to imagine different aspects of their lives as if they were very confident. They explore this image to recognise how they would speak, feel, note the response of others and create improvements at work and home. I ask them to practise this experience during self-hypnosis on a daily basis until the attitudes and feelings emerge in reality.

Many deep trance phenomena occur in the normal waking state. Ask witnesses to a traffic accident what they saw and there will be many different versions – hallucination; how often do we go upstairs for something and forget what it was – amnesia; we focus so strongly on an intense drama we do not move – catalepsy; we are involved in a funny film and do not notice our toothache – analgesia.

The benefits of hypnosis are that we can specifically create some of these phenomena and tailor them to help the patient. Parallels between the patients' experience in trance and their experiences in life are used to overcome difficulties.

7

The Initial Interview

*To make an end is to make a beginning. The end is where
we start from.*

T. S. Eliot

Many patients have told me how nervous they were during
the first consultation. This is perfectly normal as they were
talking about intimate subjects with a stranger who may
have used a technique they didn't understand.

I would like to list some aspects of therapy to reassure you
about what is involved. I will describe them firstly from a
patient's and then a therapist's point of view.

Patient's Point of View

Motivation

One of the most important factors necessary to resolve
problems is motivation. The more motivated you are to
achieve improvement the more likely it is to occur.

'My wife wants me to see you because I have a violent
temper' is vastly different from 'I'm so fed up with my

temper, it is ruining my life, work and relationships. I'm really determined to do something about it, that's why I'm here.'

It is not only the need but the desire which provides energy for change. People who seek help for cancer will travel miles, have unpleasant treatments, put off other appointments, etc. to achieve a cure. They make it the number one priority in their life. Many patients seeking therapy are in conflict as to whether to proceed or not so their motivation is diluted.

Time

When you choose to see a therapist is important. You need to be ready to put in time and effort. Often people come to see me and they are not ready for what is involved to deal with their problems and take responsibility for change. It is a little like reading a self-help book such as this one. You may read it then put it away, making no use of the advice. Some time later when you re-read it the advice 'clicks' and you put the techniques into practice.

Joe's wife rang me to make an appointment for him to see me about his smoking. When he arrived he was very negative throughout the consultation inferring he had only come because his wife insisted.

He cancelled the second appointment and I did not hear from him until a year later when he rang me to arrange another session.

'Doctor, my father has just died of lung cancer. He smoked 40 cigarettes a day. I'm really keen to stop now', he said at the start of the consultation.

This time Joe did follow directions and was able to stop smoking because the time was right for him.

Making the call

The next step along the therapeutic pathway is making an appointment. I can reassure you that everyone is nervous about the first appointment. I have been there myself so I speak from experience. Therapists have different ways of making appointments. Some require a doctor's referral, some take the message themselves, some have secretaries, some send out questionnaires. It is reasonable to ask any questions you may have about the session – cost, time, what the therapist believes will happen, etc., but it is unlikely that any therapeutic advice will be given before the therapist knows more about you and your problem.

Initial meeting

During the first consultation you will have a number of senses on high alert. You will be looking at the therapist's body language and noticing a variety of things that you like or dislike. Your instinct will tell you about him without any logical thinking involved. Your feelings will be giving you messages. Your own emotions of anxiety and concern will be influencing you. Your thoughts will be racing with questions and self-doubts.

It is important during the first session that you develop a feeling of trust for the therapist. This is important as you may be exploring areas you would not willingly discuss with everyone. You also need to develop confidence that this person is competent, that he understands you as an individual, that you are both on the same wavelength and that he feels right to deal with your problem.

First impressions

It is likely that you will feel a little confused at the start as you are sharing something very personal and receiving comments from a stranger. Your mind and emotions are doing many things in this first session (which will generally be an hour long) both in dealing with your fears as well as assessing him. Rely on your instincts and if it doesn't feel right for you then it isn't.

Realise that the first session is as much an assessment as a therapy session. If it feels right then it is worthwhile lowering barriers as time goes by, but keeping the right to raise them if necessary.

Your aim

It is important to have an aim. Many therapy situations falter because there was no original goal stated in the first interview. It needs to be specific not something like 'I want to be happy' or 'I want everyone to like me'. It also needs to be attainable. 'I would like to overcome my panic attacks so I can go to the cinema without fear.'

Having both you and the therapist aware of this aim provides a track upon which therapy is directed. It may well be that other goals surface with time and these can then be assessed and addressed.

Your history

A history of you and your problem will be taken because it is the *person* receiving the treatment not the problem. There may be obvious causes or it may require the therapist's expertise to decide what aspects of your history to explore. Childhood experiences can be relevant as unresolved emotions often surface as symptoms in later life.

Establishing rapport

If you wish to understand aspects of yourself or the therapy
it is important that the rapport is good enough for you to be
able to ask your therapist any questions about anything.

What to expect

Hypnosis will not always be used in the first session as the
therapist needs to understand the problems, the aims and
you as an individual in order to formulate a plan for therapy.
If hypnosis is used he may employ some of the techniques
mentioned in later chapters. The basic aim is to teach you
to relax and guide you into a trance so that the conscious–
unconscious communication can be utilised to deal with
your problem.

You will go into deeper trances each time you use
hypnosis so do not be concerned in the first visit if nothing
appears to be happening.

Homework

At the end of the session the therapist may give you 'homework' to gain experience of the theories discussed during the
session. He may give you an hypnosis tape to reinforce the
work he has started. If you have gone into a trance state you
will be very relaxed when you leave, but you should be in
control of all your faculties and able to drive if you need to.

Another very important factor determining the successful outcome of therapy, apart from motivation, is your
ability to put time and effort into the homework suggested.
Unfortunately, so many patients come to see me saying, 'I'll
do anything to overcome this problem' and I ask them to

listen to a tape three times a week and they return saying they did not have the time.

Therapist's Point of View

The session should include the following aims:

1. To enable the patient to develop trust and confidence in you and your ability.
2. To give positive messages about the patient and his problem.
3. To be aware of body language and unconscious messages, and give attentive listening at all times.
4. To explain the basics of hypnosis and answer any questions however trivial they may seem.
5. To treat the patient as an individual, rather than a symptom, and respect the patient as such.
6. To proceed at a pace that is suitable to the patient.
7. To be supportive and understanding rather than superior and directive.
8. To demystify hypnosis rather than promote it as a magic wand that solves everything.
9. To understand the patient's viewpoint and know where they are coming from.
10. To keep the aim in mind so that therapy is in that direction even though it may be diverted from time to time.
11. To give hope where it is appropriate as this is a great vehicle to promote motivation.

Follow Your Intuition

It is difficult to describe individual consultations as they vary greatly depending on the patient, the therapist and the problem. It is important that the patient believes in his right to express concerns and doubts, and that both the patient and therapist are honest with their attitudes and statements.

As a general rule relying on your intuition is a good guide as to whether things are going well for you or not. I know it is difficult if you lose confidence and have trouble deciding anything, let alone if the therapist is suitable or not. Deep down you will have a 'gut reaction' and it is useful to rely on this for guidance.

There should be very little to be worried about during a therapy session. Frightening emotions from the past may come to consciousness but they should be dealt with in a way that is healing and supportive. Just as taking out a splinter causes pain, so releasing conflicts can be upsetting, but as the finger heals after the splinter is removed, so does the mind after the emotion is released.

As a rule hypnotherapy is a much shorter treatment than many of the other 'talking therapies' such as analysis. The number of sessions depends on many things and it is wise to discuss this with the therapist so you both have an understanding. Some therapists suggest six sessions and then reassess progress to see if more are required.

Above all, realise that the consultations are to help you with your problem. Make sure you talk about your needs and concerns so you are playing a positive role in the direction your therapy is going.

For whatever reason you seek therapy, an underlying focus of the therapist will be to help you learn about yourself (conscious, unconscious and emotions), so that you can resolve conflicts and gain control of your life.

PART 2

Learning About the Mind

8

Close Your Eyes
and See

*We have three eyes; two look outwards to see the outward
world; one looks inwards to see ourselves as we really are.*

Brian Roet

Recently, I was in charge of a seminar on stress management
and asked for a volunteer to come to the front so I could
demonstrate how to communicate with the unconscious
mind. A woman of about 40 volunteered, saying she would
like to find out why she was persistently critical of herself.
She had a voice in her head telling her she should do better
no matter what she did. I asked her to sit comfortably, close
her eyes and learn whose voice it was.

In a few seconds she opened her eyes in surprise, 'I can see
him. It's my father. He was always judging me but I didn't
know it was his voice causing all this trouble.'

The woman closed her eyes and saw. It took only a
moment for her to understand an internal mechanism that
had troubled her for years. I am not saying the voice
stopped, but she certainly learnt something that would allow
her to work on the problem and in time, perhaps, diminish
her critical voice. I find it really surprising that sometimes it

takes only seconds to learn a great deal by the simple action of closing your eyes and focusing internally.

I compare this experience to someone visiting a coral reef. From the boat you can see the water, the beach and the sky but if you put on a mask and snorkel, a whole new world of coloured fish and coral opens up to you.

So it is with the unconscious. It is there awaiting you. It is available if you take the time and effort to have a quiet period with your eyes closed, focusing internally, and being in a passive rather than active mode. You can see with your eyes closed, the visions are in your mind, but they are vivid and feel real just as dreams do.

In the same seminar a man asked if he could learn about an angry feeling that had troubled him for years. He came to the front, sat next to me and I asked him to explain further.

'It often happens when someone does something I don't like, especially at work. I get so angry I want to kick something and often I have to leave the room in case I hurt the person involved.'

'Where in your body do you get the feeling?'

'I don't know.'

As he said this, his hand went to his chest, an unconscious action pointing to where the feeling was.

'Is it in your chest, do you think?'

'I suppose it could be.'

'Why don't we explore it and learn what we can. Close your eyes and imagine you are in your chest. When you are there let me know.'

A minute later he nodded his head.

'Imagine you have the angry feeling and when you have it, nod your head.'

A minute later he nodded his head again.

'Have a look at the feeling and tell me what you see.'

A little while later he spoke slowly, 'It is black and ugly I don't know how to describe it.'

'When you have an experience that causes this black, ugly feeling, what feeling would you rather have instead?'

He was quiet for a little while.

'I'd like a smiley face, like a girl I knew who was very positive.'

'Good. Put that face in your chest and tell me how it feels.'

After a while, he said, 'It feels better. I feel lighter and more comfortable. The black, ugly thing has shrunk and is very small now and the face is large and feels good.'

'Could you spend some time making sure you build up the face and decrease the black, ugly thing?'

'Yes.'

'Good. Take your time and when you are ready come back and join the group.'

This man was able to learn that, as a result of closing his eyes and seeing something that he was unaware of, he would be able to make an improvement to his life. It was as if he had put on a mask and snorkel and was delighted at the coral reef that met his eyes when he looked underwater.

Many people go through life without ever giving them-selves the time to close their eyes and see. They are too busy doing things. Their lives are so hectic they feel it would be a waste of time if they were not actively performing some function, whether in a relationship, at home or at work.

Yet it is so simple. There are not many things in this life easier than sitting quietly and closing your eyes. It is as if 'no task' becomes 'a great task'. Most people put this exercise on their agenda to do when everything is done. And it never is.

In a way it is like an essential vitamin we need to take daily. Many find the taking of a tablet can be fitted into their busy schedule but 20 minutes' quiet time is too much to ask.

If a problem has a psychological component no one can fix it for you. It is not like a surgical problem where removal gives a cure. The answers lie within and you can be helped by a guide or therapist to find them. Your resources are already there, it is the task of the guide to help you unearth them.

Perhaps it would be better for you to put down this book now and have some quiet time exploring your inner thoughts, rather than continuing to read.

Insight and sight look in completely opposite directions and hence discover vastly different panoramas.

9

The Mind as a Computer and its Protective Role

We are generally the better persuaded by the reasons we discover ourselves than by those given to us by others.

Pascal

If we regard the mind as a computer it helps us understand some of our actions, and also some of the difficulties in achieving our aims. A child growing up feeds experiences into the mind computer. All this information is used as the software for future experiences.

To the baby and young child the most powerful force is that of survival. This is an internal force inherited from the cave man, and prehistoric animals before him. So the computer acknowledges, and underlines in red, any experiences which may put survival in jeopardy. Those situations are stored in a special compartment. They are magnified to ensure protection is at a maximum.

It is as if a wealthy man has had his house broken into and something of importance stolen. He fits a burglar alarm which helps for a while, but when he is burgled again, he installs an alarm that is so sensitive the slightest movement triggers it off. All goes well, until he forgets to switch it on and he is nearly burgled again.

He decides to leave the alarm on all the time. His thoughts, actions and dreams are entirely concerned with ensuring his safety. The alarm is successful in guarding him from burglary, but he cannot move freely without setting it off. He cannot have any pets, his windows are sealed so the breeze cannot move the curtains, and he remains in one room so as not to disturb the alarm. An extreme and absurd story but it illustrates the protective role our computer minds play in limiting us in adult life.

The young child learns how important it is not to upset his mother. She is his lifeline – if she is upset she may cut him off. The guarding function of the mind says, 'Don't do that, don't think this, don't feel that', in order to screen the child from rejection and desertion. When parents are in control these devices may be life-saving and very successful. The child restricts his thoughts, feelings and actions in a similar way to an animal which remains motionless when caught in a snare, realising every movement may bring great pain.

The programme of the mind's computer is made up of experience upon experience, fear upon fear and these become magnified as time goes by. The guardian role of the mind uses these enlarged fears to shield us from present situations. Often these protective devices are not required and are in fact limiting and disturbing in themselves.

Imagine a young child wandering off at a picnic and becoming lost temporarily in the woods. He is frightened and cold and misses his mum. Let us assume there are two alternative mothers who find him.

Mother A shows her relief and love by cuddling him, reassuring him everything will be all right, that it was not his fault but he must be wary of wandering off in the future. Although still part of his memory, his fears are minimised; he feels little guilt or rejection.

Mother B finds him, and her anxiety and concern are shown in anger and disapproval. She cries and screams at him – how stupid he is to wander off and cause so much trouble. 'You could have died of cold and think how Mummy would feel then.' She is not only criticising his action but also criticising the child himself. That child will have fear, guilt and pain built into his computer so that any future similar experience will bring the guardian angel in to restrict him and prevent the pain occurring again. Any experiences in the future involving independence or exploration may be severely curtailed.

The mind acts rather as a radar does, screening each second we live and comparing it with the past, noting any similarity to previous danger areas and bringing in protective devices if needed. The problem with the protective devices in the mind is that they can still operate to keep a child safe long after childhood has passed.

This blocking of abilities in the adult, when implemented by fear or guilt, is a very powerful force. When these feelings play a great role in a *child's* learning experiences he will find them difficult to overcome when tackling life's normal problems in *adulthood*. Even though he may have had many positive experiences to boost his self-confidence, the protective radar picks up the fear and guilt much more easily than the pride and confidence from successful actions.

Toby is 40, a businessman, married, successful. However, he has trouble talking to people, relating, expressing himself. When he meets strangers, he knows what he wants to say but he seems to freeze and smile in an embarrassed way. He feels foolish and thinks people regard him as dumb. He avoids these situations because they are too painful.

After a few sessions using hypnosis and teaching Toby self-hypnosis, he recognised two parts in his mind advising him how to behave. One part, the adventurous one, said, 'Go ahead, say what you think, it will be well received.' The other part, the protective one, then said to him, 'Don't say that, they will all laugh at you.'

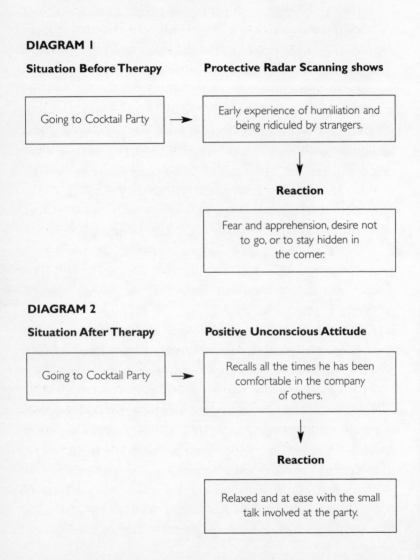

DIAGRAM 1

Situation Before Therapy   **Protective Radar Scanning shows**

| Going to Cocktail Party | → | Early experience of humiliation and being ridiculed by strangers. |

Reaction

| Fear and apprehension, desire not to go, or to stay hidden in the corner. |

DIAGRAM 2

Situation After Therapy   **Positive Unconscious Attitude**

| Going to Cocktail Party | → | Recalls all the times he has been comfortable in the company of others. |

Reaction

| Relaxed and at ease with the small talk involved at the party. |

He learnt to join the two parts into a three-way discussion on how he should act – he had a say in things. Gradually he allowed the guardian protector, which was still treating him as a child, to go off duty. With time and experience he became more comfortable in company and chose not to avoid it as he had done previously.

Toby's reaction to an intended cocktail party could have been represented 'Before Treatment' as in Diagram 1 opposite. The cocktail party triggered a scanning by the protective radar which recalled previous experiences that were painful. It is interesting that this device is so specialised it does not connect with experiences that have been successful. Toby then felt the fear from the past and acted reflexively, without conscious control, to stay in a corner and wish he was home.

After treatment Toby could focus on positive experiences he could recall in order to realise he possessed all the requirements to enjoy the party. He had learnt, through repeated self-hypnosis, to 're-brainwash' his mind to believe he was a normal healthy person the same as all the others at the party and he could enjoy it in the same way that they were (see Diagram 2).

Hypnosis is a useful mechanism to re-programme the mind's computer and look at early experiences from the distance of the present. It is also helpful to feed in positive experiences and abilities, to help the unconscious realise that the protective mechanism is no longer needed in such strength. Hypnosis can remove the unnecessary blocks placed on emotions and abilities many years previously. Removing these blocks allows freedom to 'be yourself', to be able to accept your feelings as your own, without associated guilt, to react to situations without fear and insecurity, but with the confidence to use the powers that are available.

Two of these blocks are *guilt* and *fear*.

Guilt is one of the least beneficial emotions; doing things or not doing things because of a guilty feeling is most restrictive. The majority of inter-reactions due to guilt do not provide growth for either the giver or receiver. It is an emotion brought about by parental displeasure, and continued in the mind as its most powerful negative force. Many people who have had 'guilt-making' parents go through life feeling guilty about saying, feeling, thinking even the most trivially assertive things, even guilty for being alive. They have lived with this guilt for so long it has become part of them and they may even feel guilty without it. Any attempt by them to gain access to their adult resources, used to wend their way through life, is stopped by the all-pervading guilt.

Fear of what may happen is an extremely limiting force, preventing people from reaching their potential. Fear learnt at an early age can be pervasive through the years and interferes with the freedom and enjoyment so easily obtained by those who grew up with security.

Often fear and guilt are completely illogical and require a double approach: re-training the mind and having practical experience to lay down new beliefs.

These two approaches require risk-taking and new learning and are complementary to each other. Often the therapist will give 'homework' to provide practical support to the theoretical discussions occurring during the sessions.

Using the metaphor of the computer it is important to have up-to-date and effective software running our thoughts and emotions.

10

The Language of the Unconscious

We make many mistakes in life, feeling when we ought to think, and thinking when we should be feeling.

Brian Roet

As hypnosis is 'communicating with the unconscious and updating it', it is important to learn about the language of the unconscious in order to understand how hypnotherapy works.

The unconscious is dominant in both a trance and dream states, so by studying dreams we can learn a great deal about methods used by the unconscious to convey messages to the conscious. Dreams use stories and symbols. The stories are relevant to what is happening in daily life and recount messages we can absorb without waking up. Both stories and symbols represent events, attitudes and behaviour and by interpreting these representations we come to understand ourselves and the way we act.

Joseph's wife had breast cancer. She was receiving chemo-therapy. The last treatment was to be on the following week and he would not know the outcome for some time. Joseph had a dream the night before seeing me:

'I am in a boat being tossed around by a stormy sea. There is no rudder on the boat and I don't know where I am going. The sea calms down but I still have no idea of my destination.'

The dream is telling Joseph about his personal situation. It is using symbols and metaphors parallel to his conscious experience.

The language of the conscious mind involves thoughts, reasoning, analysis and facts whilst the unconscious uses feelings, metaphors, symbolism, symptoms and literal language.

Some researchers believe our unconscious is related to an ancient part of the mind evolved from animals. Not having the complexity of human vocabulary, animals use body language to convey vital messages. It is thought that many of our involuntary reflexes come from these origins. Blushing may be the remnant of facial reactions in animals – elephants waving their ears to frighten predators, the hair on a dog rising to give the message of aggression.

Metaphors

When we suffer from symptoms these may in fact be unconscious messages or metaphors about conflicts and unresolved emotions from the past. As the unconscious does not use words it may use bodily symptoms or 'body language' to let us know about out-of-date processes.

Liza had been vomiting once or twice a day for the last two years. She was an anxious 30-year-old who had many other problems and difficulties in her life. She was referred to me by her doctor who was worried about her vomiting and weight loss.

Over a number of sessions I learnt about Liza and started to understand her approach to life – her strengths and fears, her relationship problems and her attitude to the world.

I decided to use hypnosis to learn more about her vomiting. After inducing a trance I asked her some questions.

I discovered she felt that she had to vomit every day. A voice situated at the back of her head was telling her she must. She said it was 'the inner voice'. We found out it was a woman so I asked Liza why she wanted her to be sick.

'She says it's a punishment for being pregnant and having a termination three years ago.'

'Did you have morning sickness then?'

'Yes.'

I left her to sit quietly for a few minutes to digest what we had discussed. Suddenly as if a thought came to her, she said, 'She's just like my mother.'

At that stage Liza opened her eyes and came out of the trance. 'I never thought of that. How it fits in. My mother was always criticising me and now the voice is doing exactly the same.'

We spent the next few sessions discussing what Liza had discovered and gradually her vomiting stopped as she became consciously aware of the underlying mechanism that had been causing it.

Liza's story illustrates how the unconscious uses symptoms and metaphors to deal with unresolved conflicts. Her mother made her feel guilty about the pregnancy and termi- nation. This guilt was transferred to 'the inner voice', a metaphor for her mother. The form of punishment involved was related to the 'crime'. Once Liza was able to bring to her conscious mind what was happening via hypnosis, she was able to overrule the internal voice and forgive herself for what happened three years previously.

Decoding metaphors

Hypnosis is a very useful tool for decoding metaphors and symbolism used by the unconscious. The symptoms we have are often literal representations of an unconscious process. The concept 'symptoms are messages' helps us understand just how the unconscious mind influences our lives.

Claude had diarrhoea on and off for months. He saw a number of doctors and had blood tests, a barium enema and a scan. The tests were normal but Claude was still worried. He was a 50-year-old businessman who had been promoted six months before I saw him.

He was referred to me by his GP but was very sceptical that I could help. 'I'm only coming to see you because my GP and wife insist. They think I'm loopy but I know this is a real problem and I can't see how hypnosis could be of any use.'

'You may well be correct, Claude, but there is often a strong connection between the mind and the body, and as the tests are negative it may be worthwhile exploring that area.'

'Well, there is nothing wrong in my life except my work and that is giving me the shits.'

My ears pricked up at Claude's comment. Was the unconscious telling me of a connection between his work and diarrhoea? Claude agreed to see me for four visits and if there was no improvement he would stop therapy.

On the second visit I showed Claude how to go into a trance and made a tape for him to play each day. The words on the tape were about the bowel and how it felt about his promotion.

During his third visit Claude commented that perhaps his GP was right and that the stress of the job may be related to his diarrhoea. We continued to discuss ways of looking at his promotion that might be less stressful.

At the fourth visit, even though his diarrhoea had not improved very much, he agreed to continue the sessions as he was feeling less tense after the relaxation exercises I had taught him.

Claude came to see me for three months and during that time decided he didn't want to be promoted. He negotiated with his firm to have his old job back and was much happier with this outcome – so was his bowel.

The initial clue that helped me focus on Claude's problem was the unconscious message that his work was 'giving him the shits'.

Messages for the unconscious

Hypnotherapy often makes use of metaphor to alter the perspective of the unconscious, to give messages on a deeper level so that change can take place. As this method avoids conscious analysis it also circumvents resistance to change, as the message is being received beyond conscious awareness.

If a patient is frightened of taking risks and this fear is causing problems in his life I may tell the following story when he is in a trance:

In the last war there was fighting between the Japanese and Americans in the Philippines. In 1945, when the war ended, Americans were sent into the jungle to tell the Japanese soldiers to surrender. Over the following weeks soldiers gave themselves up and were sent back to Japan. Over the following months, however, one soldier, believing it was a trick did not come out and fired on anyone who tried to make him.

This soldier stayed in the jungle for 30 years until 1975 constantly refusing to come out in case he was humiliated. He only emerged when the Emperor wrote on an official document that he would be pardoned and he was ordered to surrender. The soldier later toured Japan as a national hero. He took 30 years to overcome his fear and was only able to take a risk when he saw the document from the Emperor.

Such a story has messages for the unconscious. It is sometimes necessary to take a risk; often the things we fear are not present when we face them; it is a pity to waste one's life unnecessarily and when you do face your fears you reap a great reward.

The following is another therapeutic metaphor I tell patients who are stuck in their ways:

A woman (or man depending on the patient) lived in the jungle as did her parents and grandparents. Following family custom she would leave her hut in the morning and walk along a track to a swamp. She would stay most of the day by the swamp and return home in the evening. This is what her parents had done all their lives.

One day she thought, 'This is a boring life, why don't I do something else. But the jungle is so dense and I don't know any other track so I'd better continue going to the swamp.' But the thought wouldn't go away and it grew stronger and stronger until one night she said to herself, 'Tomorrow I'm going to take my machete and carve a new path in the jungle. I'm not sure what I'll find but at least I'll have a try.'

The next morning she got up early and went in the opposite direction and started hacking at the jungle with her machete. It was hard, hot work; she got many scratches and did not proceed very far before she was exhausted and went back to her hut. She slept well that night due to her physical tiredness and excitement at the new venture. Each morning she continued hacking into the jungle and felt so much better than before.

After many days of hard work she noticed light ahead and worked harder with her machete. Eventually she came out onto a beautiful lagoon surrounded by dazzling white sand. She ran down the beach and threw herself into the clear blue water. She saw wonderful coloured fish swimming around, and dolphins too. In the distance were islands and she could see people in canoes. She was so excited she swam there all day and returned to her hut happier than she had ever been.

Every day she went to the lagoon and swam. Some days she caught fish, other days she lay on the sand. After some weeks her neighbours from the other islands came to visit and invited her to their homes and her life was full of joy and company.

One day she decided to visit the swamp just to remind herself how life used to be. She smiled to herself when she discovered that the pathway was now over-grown by the jungle and ran down to her beach to tell her friends.

Many hypnotherapists use therapeutic metaphors during hypnosis to help patients overcome conflicts. The stories act on two levels and are not personally challenging. Fables, proverbs, poetry and music all communicate on an unconscious level, bypassing conscious analysis, their message being received on a deeper, emotional level.

I have in my consulting room a small tube made of fabric called a Chinese Finger Prison. The fabric is woven in such a way that if the tube is pulled from either end it gets narrower.

I ask a patient to put a finger from each hand into the ends of the tube. I then ask them to try and get their fingers out. As they pull, the tube becomes tighter around their fingers. If they push their fingers together the tube loosens and they can extract them. The symbolic message is not to try too hard as it only makes things worse.

Sometimes the patient and I work out a suitable metaphor together to prevent him going round in circles without a resolution. Patients often complain that they tackle the problem like a dog with a bone, never letting it go, and being exhausted in the process.

Michael was such a patient. A 35-year-old bachelor working as a computer consultant, he had been involved in a number of relationships but never found the right woman.

Then he met Jean. She was beautiful, in love with him, and wanted to marry. The only problem was that she could also be jealous, had a terrible temper, lied constantly and was forever criticising him.

Michael came to see me looking tired and haggard. 'I've not slept well for the past month trying to decide whether to marry Jean or not.'

We discussed his feelings and also the reality of the situation, but Michael was torn between being with beautiful Jean and the suffering that might cause. At the end of each session he was no closer to a decision, so when he came for the third visit I suggested we leave Jean out of the situation and find a metaphor which might be helpful.

Michael thought for a long time then said, 'I've always wanted a house with a lovely big room where I could entertain, play my stereo and relax. That is like the part of Jean I love. If I imagine this beautiful house surrounded by apartments overlooking my garden that would represent the negative aspects of Jean.'

I agreed that he had created a very useful metaphor and asked him to go into a trance and imagine living in this special house with the noisy neighbours. Michael sat very still for about ten minutes then opened his eyes and said, 'It wouldn't work, it just wouldn't work. I wouldn't enjoy my room or entertaining because of the outside influence. I can make a decision about Jean now even though I will be sad to lose her. In fact I'm surprised I found it so difficult to see things as they actually are.'

Symbolism

In dreams the unconscious demonstrates how symbols are used to give messages – an animal may be an emotion, a cigar a penis, underwater the unconscious. Hypnosis makes use of symbolism in many ways.

In Eric Berne's book *Games People Play* (Ballantine, 1996), he discusses the three roles we can play in a relationship – parent, adult, child. He describes the attitudes and behaviour of each of these components.

As children we behave like a child – someone with no power, dependent on adults for survival. A parent takes a superior role directing the child on a daily basis. There are good parents – those who love, support and respect their children – and bad parents – critical, blaming, undermining their child's confidence.

As the child grows to adulthood he retains a great deal of his childhood learning in his unconscious. In many situations he reverts to childhood behaviour involving fear, guilt or anger. We could say the symbolic child within has taken control in these times.

The parental role in our unconscious is gleaned from the myriad experiences involving interaction with parents. All too often we 'ingest' our parents' attitudes and continue them into adulthood as if we are directed internally by the symbolic parent inside. Thus we become self-critical if we were criticised in childhood; in hypnosis this 'critical parent' residing in the unconscious can be addressed in order to reduce his influence and allow the patient to become a self-determining adult.

The aim of using parent–child symbolism is to encourage the patient to let go of out-of-date parts that are controlling him and take on the responsible role of the adult.

Emotions

The unconscious uses emotions as its main form of influence (see Chapter 21). They are such powerful forces that our conscious is held hostage in many situations where we would like to be in control.

Guilt, shame, fear, anger, sadness, all take over our attitudes and behaviour, in spite of our logical minds. They prevent other parts of the mind working in a normal, healthy manner. Phrases like frozen with fear, stricken by grief, exploding with anger, all demonstrate the powerful force emotions have on our lives.

In hypnosis it is important to focus on the 'feeling' component of any experience, as this is likely to be the cause of the symptom. Regression to childhood is used to explore unresolved conflicts and discover how the child felt – not thought – about any traumatic experience.

It is the emotion stored in the unconscious that causes problems, emotion that is unresolved and is still active although out of date. Learning about these emotions, and freeing them from their time warp, is an integral part of hypnotherapy.

Control

One of the threads running through our lives is the need to be in control. This is more important with some than with others. The need is exemplified in many symptoms and behaviour.

People with phobias – agoraphobia, claustrophobia, fear of flying, of insects, birds, mice, often have an underlying feeling they are not in control in certain situations.

Relationship difficulties, panic attacks, blushing, bowel problems, public speaking, performance anxiety, all focus on the need for control.

- 'I'm terrified on motorways. I panic in case I can't get off at the right exit.'
- 'If I go to the theatre I need to sit on the aisle so I know I can leave at any time.'
- 'I'm frightened of meeting strangers as I may blush and what would they think of me?'

- 'I run a mile from birds, I never know in which direction they may fly.'

If the underlying need is to be in control then life is difficult as the world is a changing place. These needs (and fears) are coming from the unconscious which is apparent from the opening statement, 'I know [conscious] that mice are harmless but I feel [unconscious] petrified if I think one is in the room.' The message in this case is 'As I don't know where the mice will run, I will be out of control if there is one in the room.'

Techniques used to help such situations need to involve the unconscious and provide a message that it is *safe* to fly, be with mice, go to the theatre, etc.

The causes for the underlying need to be in control may be:

1. Childhood indoctrination by parents with comments such as, 'Don't get your feet wet, you'll catch your death of cold'; 'Don't swim out too far or you will drown'; 'Don't get too excited or it will end in tears'; 'Don't run too fast or you'll fall and break your leg'. The underlying message of such comments is, 'The world is a dangerous place and you must stay in control to avoid disaster.'

2. Often people have experiences where they were not in control and something terrible happened. The unconscious stores that memory and links it with a need to be in control for survival.

Sometimes patients who come for therapy state firmly that they do not want hypnosis as they need to be in control. I talk at some length about their lives and the fact that they are consulting me because they are out of control. Even the excessive need to be in control indicates they are not in control but being controlled by the excessive need. I also explain that if hypnosis is suitable for their condition it could be used to help them gain control; that they are not out of control in the hypnotic state; that a combination of conscious and unconscious abilities is being used and if they need to come back to full consciousness, they will do so immediately. The conscious mind acts as a guardian and will take over if necessary.

A patient was in a deep trance recently when we heard footsteps on the stairs to my room. In a second he was wide awake and alert and when I opened the door I found someone had mistaken my consulting room for another office. Even though my patient was deeply hypnotised and 'far away' his conscious mind was alert enough to bring him out of the trance when required.

Colin was 30 when he came to see me. He had black moods that came from nowhere and he was worried about feeling low and depressed for much of the time.

His childhood was fraught with parental fighting and arguments. His mother and father were alcoholics and life in the home for him and his two sisters was full of fear and uncertainty. He had, however, managed to hold down a good job and had a long-term relationship with a girl whom he loved.

Over a number of consultations I noticed Colin saying 'should' a great deal, and he talked about how upset he became if things did not go as he anticipated – even getting a cold – I get very upset. I want to be healthy, I don't want a blocked nose and I feel angry and low until it has gone away.'

'What are the components of the cold that upset you, Colin?' I asked.

He thought for quite a while then said, 'It is something placed on me. I'm not ready for it. I don't want it.'

After a pause I asked, 'Do you think that bears any similarity to the things that happened at home when you were a child?'

Colin slowly reflected. 'Yes. You are right. It was like that then. I was never in control and I hated it. Funny you should say that because often when I feel low those three things are part of what is happening.'

In a way the feeling of anger and depression Colin had with a cold was, metaphorically, a reflection of his childhood experience and a symbol of the influence his alcoholic parents had on him.

It was something placed on him. He was not ready for it. He did not want it.

Colin and I worked with this revelation and in time he was able to let go of the effect of his childhood to a large degree and reduce his emotional swings.

Another aspect of unconscious language that is fascinating is the fact that it cannot comprehend negative attitudes. It does not understand 'not' so it will not process it. Ask someone 'not to think of your nose' and they will immediately think of their nose either:

- because in order not to do something the mind has to do it first in order to know what it is *not* to do; or
- because negative words are not processed by the mind.

It is common to hear people using negative comments about themselves in order to improve. 'Don't be such a fool',

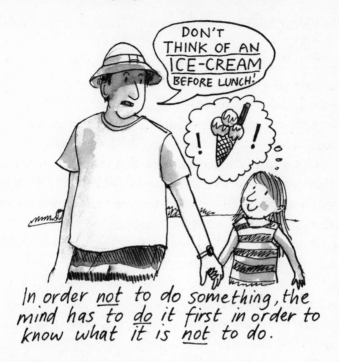

In order _not_ to do something, the mind has to _do_ it first in order to know what it is _not_ to do.

is interpreted by the unconscious mind as 'Do be a fool.' 'I mustn't stay awake tonight as I've got a busy day tomorrow.' The unconscious hears, 'I must stay awake tonight.'

This is especially important with affirmations (see Chapter 4), phrases we tell ourselves in order to achieve improvements. Such phrases require positive words rather than double negatives – 'I feel good' rather than 'I will not feel bad'.

Jenny was 14. She came to see me because she bit her nails and wished to stop. We discussed what methods she had tried already and she told me: 'I've been bribed by Mum with money but that didn't work; I've worn gloves but I took them off to bite my nails; we have painted a bitter substance on my nails but I sucked that off; I said to myself a hundred times a day "I must not bite my nails" and that didn't help.'

We chatted about many things and I asked her to imagine how the poor nails felt trying to grow, then being bitten off by her teeth.

She thought they must feel terrible and I used hypnosis to have an agreement with her teeth that they would stop hurting their friends, the fingernails. I also changed her self-talk from 'I must not bite my nails' to 'I will allow my nails their right to grow'. After a few weeks she had stopped biting her nails and came to show me how nice they looked and how proud she was that her teeth and her nails were best friends.

We can see from analysing unconscious communication that it is a complex process involving many components lacking in our rational thoughts. Just as we may have difficulty learning a new language so we may find it difficult to understand and accept the way the unconscious influences our attitudes and behaviour.

Being aware that there are three dominant components working in the depths of our minds – symbolism, metaphor and emotion – will ensure we are on the right pathway to learning more about unconscious influences and improving the balance between the two parts of our minds, the conscious and unconscious.

11

The Importance of Perspectives

The marvellous thing about a joke with a double meaning is that it can only mean one thing.

Ronnie Barker

Our perspective on an experience plays a major role in how we feel and react to it; hypnosis can play a major role in improving this reaction.

Take, for instance, the response people have to an oyster. From different points of view it could be seen as:

- alive
- tasty
- slippery
- nauseating
- expensive
- a reminder of a previously eaten bad oyster, etc.

All these points of view are factually correct, but each will lead to a different response. If we regard oysters as tasty we may order them in a restaurant; if we have previously eaten a bad oyster and suffered the consequences we may avoid them; if we think of them as alive we may be horrified at something wriggling as it slipped down our throat.

The topic I wish to discuss is not so much oysters but the influence our attitude has on our lives. Every situation has two components:

1. the actual situation
2. our perspective, viewpoint or attitude about it.

On a great many occasions we are unable to alter the situation but it is always possible to have a different attitude towards it and different emotions about it. Our beliefs have evolved from life's experiences and are not rigid unless we make them so.

Because the hypnotic state increases our suggestibility, it is a useful tool to improve our perspectives if they are causing problems. Many painful emotions are caused by attitudes forged in the flame of the past, beyond our conscious control, out of date and inappropriate for the present situation. We often lose sight of the fact that we are being manipulated by our own points of view and not by reality.

John was a keen skier. A year before he consulted me he had been skiing at dusk and narrowly missed a large tree that appeared out of the gloom. This experience shocked him so much that on his next holiday he did not ski at all. He had booked a holiday for three months after his first visit to me and needed help to regain his confidence.

The facts were that John was a competent and experienced skier; his attitude was one of terror and his perspective was indelibly marked in his emotions from the near miss. The message his unconscious was constantly stating was, 'If you ski you may die, remember the tree at dusk incident.' His mind was turned to the past and my job was to help it rotate by 180° so he could view the future in a positive and realistic way.

Firstly I taught him self-hypnosis so he could learn about deep relaxation to counteract his anxiety. He practised it daily until he could put himself into a trance quickly and easily.

Next I helped him utilise this trance state to change his perspective and see pictures of a future happy John skiing safely down the slopes rather than the John of the past narrowly missing the tree. I also had him add a 'sound-track' to his internal film – a repetitious tape saying, 'I am a competent and confident skier and I will ski safely during the holiday.' I taught him to respond to the word 'skiing' with the comfortable, safe feeling associated with his future film.

During the weeks between our sessions and his holiday John spent half an hour a day changing his attitude and feelings towards skiing. A card I received some weeks later was proof that his holiday was a great success.

How do we acquire attitudes to the variety of situations we face on a daily basis?

The answer to this question lies in the unconscious. One of its jobs is to provide mechanisms for our survival. It gathers all information relating to our experiences and computes it to create a system that will protect us in future.

This has both good and bad aspects. If we touch some-thing hot, that experience is filed in the unconscious as a warning. In this way the species is protected. Problems begin when methods of protection are not regularly updated to include the abilities we learn as we grow.

If we compare life to a war, the supreme commander needs to utilise history and assess the strength of his force and the enemy's capabilities in order to determine tactics of engagement. Taking an extreme view, if only previous battles were reviewed a nuclear enemy, in theory, could be fought by soldiers wearing armour and armed with bows and arrows.

If we look at John the skier we see that the unconscious used only one experience to form a conclusion to create fear and prevent him skiing. The other factors – John's ability, his awareness following the near miss and his keenness to ski safely – were not brought into the equation when the 'defence strategy' was implemented. The past experiences that determine unconscious activity date back to early childhood. Parental influences are a main factor in causing our belief systems. Whether we were actually instructed how to think or learnt from observation, parental attitudes play a major role in how we see the world. An anxious parent radiates anxiety throughout the household; this is picked up by children with their sensitivity to the vibrations surrounding them.

It is as if we are 'brainwashed' in childhood, and if this is not in our best interests we need to 're-brainwash' ourselves in a way that is more suitable to our needs as adults. Hypnosis, as it communicates with our unconscious, is an ideal way to alter out-of-date perspectives and replace them with more appropriate ones.

The essence of improving perspectives is illustrated by the metaphor about whether the glass is half empty or half full. The fact is that the glass contains a certain amount of water; the perspective is either:

- 'Isn't it disappointing it is half empty.'
- 'Isn't it great it is half-full.'

As I have mentioned there is often no possibility of changing the facts but there is always the opportunty to alter the point of view. Just as going underwater with a mask and snorkel changes the view dramatically so we can use the creative parts of our minds in hypnosis to adjust our angle of perception.

Changing Perspective

I would like to tell you about a recent experience I had which in a way has changed how I relate to people's opinions. When involved in a discussion or argument I used to focus on who was right and who was wrong. As I was the assessor it generally meant that I believed I was right and they were wrong. About a year ago I was contemplating two views on the lottery. One view was, 'I always buy a lottery ticket, someone has got to win.' The other was, 'I never buy a lottery ticket, the chance of winning is so remote.' Both angles are valid, yet the conclusions are dramatically opposed. As I thought about this I realised something very important – *two people can have completely opposite opinions and yet both be correct.*

This was a real discovery to me, a completely new perspective on differences of opinion. Since then I have been able to be involved in heated discussions or listen to a variety of viewpoints and not focus on who is right and who is wrong. What happens now is that I have become aware of the correct opinion both adversaries are promoting, even though they are vastly different, and now I am able to acknowledge and receive opinions without the distortion of trying to assess whether they compare favourably with my own. It makes life so much easier and also more rewarding as my focus is on a completely different perspective.

The majority of letters I receive from people who have read my self-help books have a similar message: 'I really enjoyed your book, and what helped me most was reading that others have difficulties, like mine. This provided a great deal of support and made me feel so much better.'

By reading the book with its case histories the reader had changed perspective from 'I am suffering from X. No one else has this problem, therefore there must be something terribly wrong with me and it must be my fault', to 'Many people seem to have similar problems to me. I'm not on my own; I'm like others so there is nothing wrong with me as a person.'

We often attempt to make changes but we use our energies in the wrong place. The symptoms we suffer are often the *result* of problems not the *cause*. For example, many people who are stressed get a tension headache and take pills for the pain. The cause is the stress and the pain is the result of stress so time and effort need to be spent on decreasing the stress and then the headache will go away. Hypnosis may well help in such a situation.

A joke illustrating this is as follows:

A drunk was leaning against a lamppost one night searching the ground under the light.
A passer-by asks him, 'Have you lost something?'
'Yes. I've lost my wallet.'
'Where did you lose it?'
'Over there but it's too dark to look there. I can't see anything.'

Too often we look in the easiest place because we can't be bothered to get a torch and look where the solution lies. Hypnosis may well be the torch to help us find that evasive solution.

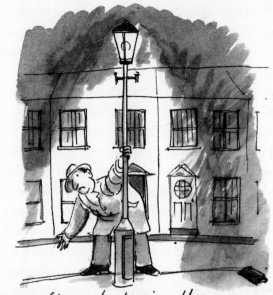

We often look in the wrong place for a solution.

There are seven unconscious systems attempting to protect us from problems. They can be recalled by the mnemonic COMPASS, each letter representing a way in which the unconscious uses past experiences to promote future actions.

C   is for conflict. One part of our mind wants to do one thing and another thinks it should do something else.

O   is for organ or body language. Chronic nausea may illustrate that 'something is making me sick' in a psychological way.

M   is for motivation. There may be some secondary
        gain from our behaviour. Our illness may achieve
        the attention that was lacking in childhood.

P   is for past experience. Traumatic experiences are
        often stored in a special part of our unconscious so
        that future events can trigger a reaction.

A   is for accepted identification. Often we identify
        with one of our parents and display behaviour or
        attitudes we have learnt through constant contact.

S   is for self-punishment. Guilt and self-punishment
        may well be the underlying factor in painful or
        disturbing symptoms.

S   is for suggestion. In childhood we receive many
        messages from authority figures. Sometimes these
        comments go into the unconscious mind as
        commands, and are adhered to as if unchangeable.

One or more of these mechanisms may well be acting to
create symptoms. Hypnosis is used to understand the cause
as well as negotiate more suitable alternatives to remove the
symptoms.

The 'Aha phenomenon'

One of the most pleasing experiences in therapy is when a
patient suddenly recognises a different way of seeing things.
It is called the 'Aha phenomenon'; a light suddenly turns on
in the mind and body language illustrates a dramatic change
has taken place. This change is often accompanied by the
comment, 'You know I've never looked at it that way before'
or 'I've never thought of it like that'. This new point of view
means that the patient will have a different attitude and
behaviour towards the situation in future. This may be

enough to solve the problem for which they have sought help.

James came to see me about his teenage son, Simon, who was forever arguing and disagreeing with his father; James felt an underlying anger and his resentment was damaging the relationship.

We discussed the ideals James held as important, his own upbringing and the attitude of his father, and it became very apparent that Simon and James were very different people whose values and aims had little in common.

My aim was to help James reframe his view of his son so he could appreciate the differences in their characters. I used hypnosis to diminish conscious resistance and contact a more receptive part of James' mind. In the trance I asked him to imagine 'two Simons': one was a wimp who followed everything his father said, had no will of his own, and would be pushed around by bosses and partners as he grew older; the other was an individual who knew his own mind, had the confidence to achieve his aims, was his own man and would forge a way through life whatever the obstacles.

James sat quietly comparing these two Simons. He remained in deep concentration for a long time and focused on his task. After he opened his eyes he was silent and thoughtful for a minute or two. When he spoke it was in a quiet and pensive voice.

'Somehow I see him differently. It is OK to do what he is doing, it will be helpful later on. I think I've been expecting too much. That was really helpful.'

When he left, James was going through the process of adjusting his view of Simon from 'difficult' to 'determined' and he needed time by himself to do this.

I didn't see James for some months until he consulted me about a completely different subject. At the end of the session I casually asked 'How is Simon these days?'

'He's fine, thanks. Doing well,' and his body language told me that the conflict had been resolved.

There is a well-known psychological puzzle called the nine dot puzzle. The task is to join the nine dots by four straight lines not taking the biro off the paper.

The answer can only be achieved by altering your view of the puzzle. In much the same way the trance state helps resolve 'unresolvable' problems by helping us to view them differently.*

---

*If you are having difficulty finding the answer to the nine dot problem, to put you out of your misery, it is on page 268.

12

Past-life Regression

*Life is all memory, except for the one present moment that
goes by you so quickly you hardly catch it going.*

Tennessee Williams

I am including a chapter on past-life regression because of
the many queries I have received over the last 20 years.
There is often a connection in people's minds between
hypnosis and past lives and there are those who are
fascinated by the concept and others who are terrified. This
has come about not only from films and books on the
subject but also from beliefs and fantasies. It is certainly
possible to use hypnosis to help people remember events
from the past. On many occasions I have enabled people to
find jewellery or money which they have hidden for safe-
keeping and subsequently forgotten the hiding place.

For many years I had two containers in my mind – one for
things I knew to be true, the other for things I thought were
false. I have now added a third one in the middle containing
things I am unsure about. Past-life regression is in this
container.

My view on this subject is that it is a very useful metaphor and I use it in therapy as such. I do not wish to validate whether the lives actually occurred or not, my main attitude is whether it helps the patient. On a number of occasions people have spontaneously regressed to a previous life when questioned about past experiences. I have made use of their 'imagination' to help them with their problem.

Sometimes the unexpected happens in a trance which cannot be explained logically.

Ruth was a 50-year-old mother of three children. She went into a trance easily and over a period of therapy described life as a Native American in the 1800s. On one occasion she talked about sitting with the elders of the tribe and being offered a 'calumet'. I had no idea what this was but transcribed as she spoke.

Being a deep subject Ruth often had no recollection of her trance experiences and when I said afterwards, 'You mentioned a word 'calumet' in your trance, what does it mean?' she told me she had no idea and had never heard of the word before. So I looked it up in the dictionary. To my amazement, there it was, 'calumet – a peace-pipe.'

At one level Ruth knew about a calumet but at a conscious level she did not.

She had never studied North American culture and would have been extremely unlikely to come into contact with such a word. Does this indicate that Ruth had a previous life as a Native American? I don't know and feel comfortable with leaving it in the 'don't know' container in my mind. It was not important for Ruth's therapy to explore that area any further.

The main message involved in past-life therapy is that the experiences in trance are similar to dreams in that they are metaphors from the unconscious. These metaphors are very powerful and can be extremely helpful in resolving troublesome conflicts. Some therapists use past-life regression as a mainstay of their therapy.

When I am questioning someone in a trance about the cause of a symptom the sequence may go something like this:

'At what age did the symptom become part of you?' – 'I've always had it.'
'Did you have it before you were ten years old?' – 'Yes.'
'Did you have it when you were born?' – 'Yes.'
'Did you have it before you were born - in the womb?' – 'Yes.'
'Did you have it in a previous life?' – 'Yes.'

And so the patient is led into a past-life experience to describe what they see. I enquire about the clothing, place, date if they know it, who they were, what they did and how the symptom was involved in their life. I may also ask how they died and if there was a previous life before that. All the time I am questioning I am looking for relevant details that have a direct connection to the present-day problem.

Joanna was terrified of water. She couldn't go swimming and showered instead of bathing. She told me she had always been frightened as a child and now at the age of 30 had decided to do something about it.

I asked her to discuss her fear with her mother and find out if there had been experiences in childhood that might be relevant or if her mother or father were frightened of water. At the next session she reported that she had always had her fear even as a small babe and her mother could not recall any instances where she had fallen into water.

In a trance she went back to a past life and recalled with great emotion an incident in the nineteenth century when she was walking her dog in the woods. She threw a stick into a pond, the dog jumped in to retrieve it and became entangled under the water. Jumping in after the dog she too became entangled and drowned.

Whilst Joanna was recounting this story she was shaking with fear and crying uncontrollably. When she came out of the trance she was exhausted.

'What a terrible experience. I had no idea that would happen. What does it mean, did I live in the past?'

'I really don't know but it may help you with your fear of water.'

We spent the next two sessions discussing Joanna's trance experience and I taught her relaxation exercises so she could allow her images to drift into the past and be disconnected from the intense emotion she had associated with them. She did lose her fear of water but this change did not occur spontaneously after her past-life experience. Other pieces of the jigsaw needed to be put into place before her fears subsided.

If we consider the things we inherit from our forefathers it makes sense that past experiences may be passed on in our genetic material. Jung talks of a 'collective unconsciousness' where the unconscious pool contains memories and experiences from our ancestors. Past-life regression may also be of this form and explained by memories handed down through the ages. The 'déjà-vu' experiences we all have from time to time may also fit in with this concept. As my main aim is to use hypnotic experiences for therapeutic benefit, it is academic whether the past life is actually 'true' or not. In therapy the focus is constantly on 'How can I help the patient to make use of this information? How can I guide him to explore this metaphor correlating it to events and attitudes that are happening in his life?', in much the same way dream interpretation is explored to understand unconscious mechanisms.

Philip, a 32-year-old artist came to see me with depression. He had been in good health most of his life apart from the depression which started two years previously. His moods had varied from 'low to black'; he had been seeing a psychiatrist and taking anti-depressants for the past three months.

During a number of consultations I taught him relaxation and ego-strengthening techniques and helped him to explore his emotions, but his condition deteriorated and I became concerned when he used terms such as, 'I can't stand it any more' and 'life isn't worth living'.

During one session in a trance he commented, 'It is like the devil side of me is taking over.'

He told me that the devil had always been there, since before he was born. When I asked him if he had had a past-life, he paused for about a minute before replying, 'Yes.'

'I was Gertrude, a barmaid, and lived in London in the 1800s. I was not married, I had no children and had a hard life stealing and cheating. I drowned myself when I was 23.'

He revealed that the devil had been in him then and caused him to do 'all the nasty things'. When I asked him what happened when he died he replied, 'It was lovely, calm and peaceful. The devil was outside me, waiting for my next body.'

He continued to describe previous lives of people who had been influenced by 'the devil' and had tragic deaths. He commented that he wished to expel the devil. I asked him if he was ready to start to do that now and he replied that he was.

For some minutes Philip sat motionless, intent on something happening inside. Then he bent forward and started pushing like a woman delivering a baby. After about three minutes he opened his eyes and sat up.

I remained silent for some minutes waiting for Philip to speak. When he did he remembered everything that had happened in the trance. 'That was amazing. What a strange experience. Do you think it is true?' I told him that I did not know.

He described the devil as being like a ball of grey gas in his stomach. When he pushed hard some came out.

I counselled Philip over the next two weeks to support him after his experience. He felt more confident and powerful and his paranoia subsided. His depression still fluctuated so he was prescribed increased anti-depressants by his psychiatrist but he never returned to the deep despair he had previously suffered.

There are books in the Further Reading section to help if you are interested in studying past-life regression. Whether real or not, past-life therapy can be very useful in providing resources for people who struggle to find causes for their symptoms.

13

Hypnosis and Psychosomatic Illness

Hope is the feeling you have that the feeling you have isn't permanent.

Jean Kerr

The word 'psychosomatic' is a combination of 'psycho' meaning mind and 'soma' meaning body. Mind–body illnesses differ from organic ones that are caused by bacteria, injury or physical disease. However, most illnesses have a psychological component. We do think and have emotions about the way we feel. In psychosomatic conditions the mind plays a major role in either causing or maintaining the problem.

One of the difficulties in our attitude towards illness is that, if the mind is involved, we tend to think it is our fault, feel guilty and believe we should fix it ourselves rather than seek professional help.

- 'I'm so ashamed of my depression. There is nothing to show for it like a plaster cast. People won't believe me when I tell them how awful I feel.'
- 'I really feel guilty wasting your time with my panic

attacks when there are other patients with real difficulties.'

Learning that psychosomatic problems are just as real and just as painful and disturbing as organic ones is important if a cure is to be achieved. No blame or guilt should be involved as the unconscious mind and body have caused the problem and it is up to the patient and therapist to resolve it.

As hypnosis is involved in helping the conscious–unconscious-body connections it follows that it can be a very useful tool in curing psychosomatic illnesses.

Sarah came to see me with chronic headaches. They had started after she hit her head on a low beam more than a year before. She needed to lie down and the pain stayed with her for several days.

A friend had told her a story about someone who developed a clot in the brain following a similar incident and Sarah started to worry. She saw her doctor who examined and reassured her, but this wasn't enough.

Her opening remark to me was, 'How can I be sure I don't have a blood clot causing this headache? The pain is real, but my GP must have thought I was imagining it as he sent me to a shrink like you.'

'You can't be sure, Sarah. All we know is that for over a year you have had headaches, all the tests have been negative and you are worried you may have a clot in your brain. Do you know anyone who had a clot on the brain?'

'Yes. An uncle. The doctors misdiagnosed his condition after a fall. They reassured him nothing was wrong and then he died three weeks later.'

'It is a year since you hurt your head so that is a little different. The likelihood is that continuing worry and muscular tension are causing the headaches. Would it be all right if I taught you hypnosis so you could reduce the headaches, or do you think they serve a purpose by keeping you aware of the possibility of a clot?'

'I'd love to lose the damn headaches but if you get rid of them with hypnosis, people would believe I was imagining them all along and I'd look a fool.'

'Well, that's a possibility, but maybe if we just talk about muscle relaxation and reducing tension people would accept that as a reasonable treatment for chronic headaches.'

Sarah and I worked together for three months. She practised self-hypnosis every day and gradually realised, at a conscious and unconscious level, that the chances of a blood clot causing problems after all this time were minimal.

Her headaches disappeared for some days, then returned but over the three months continued to decrease. She was able to reduce the 'psycho' component of her psychosomatic headaches and the 'somatic' component followed.

How do we know whether a symptom is physical or psychological? This is not an easy question and depends on the medical advice received. Many conditions are obviously organic in nature; many psychological and still others have components of both. Checking through the systems in the body it is possible to list illnesses that could be labelled psychosomatic.

Skin:	Blushing, eczema, psoriasis.
Nervous System:	Panic attacks, headaches, tics, stammering, tremors.

Digestive System:	Ulcers, irritable bowel syndrome, soiling in childhood, constipation and diarrhoea.
Respiratory System:	Asthma, chronic cough, hyperventilation.
Reproductive System:	Premature ejaculation, impotence, menstrual disorders, many sexual difficulties.
Muscles:	Back pains, cramps, muscle tension, torticollis.

It is apparent that the mind–body connection is constantly in operation causing symptoms that require attention. Often these symptoms can be regarded as a 'message to be understood', rather than a 'problem to be fixed'. Once the 'message' is decoded, the need for the mind–body system to continue the symptom is removed and it goes away.

Sometimes the message is out of date or inappropriate so the use of hypnosis is two-fold: firstly decoding the message and secondly informing the unconscious it is no longer appropriate or helpful.

Reuben was a 60-year-old engineer who had chronic insomnia. He was awake most of the night and stated that although he was very tired when he went to bed, as soon as his head touched the pillow he became wide awake. This condition had lasted for 30 years and resisted all the medication prescribed over that period.

Polish in origin, Reuben had gone to Australia after the war. For six months before the war ended he had been a Russian prisoner of war. He was sent to Siberia where he had only rags to protect him from the snow. The men slept in a large tent with three braziers burning to give minimal warmth. Reuben fought hard to be close to the fire because those some distance from the heat frequently froze to death during the night. If someone close to the fire fell asleep he would be dragged away by a colleague who took his place. Reuben made a commitment never to go to sleep as, in those circumstances, sleep meant death.

Using hypnosis I explored the possibility that the unconscious was still responding to the internal tape 'sleep means death'. I guided Reuben into a deep trance and asked the unconscious the following questions:

'Are you aware that Reuben has difficulty sleeping?'

'Yes.'

'Is this difficulty related to the situation in the tent in Siberia?'

'Yes.'

'How old is Reuben?'

'Thirty.' [The age he was during the war.]

'Do you know which country he is in?'

'Siberia.'

So the unconscious was trying to keep him alive, by keeping him awake. The work we did was to inform and update his unconscious by repeated sessions where the trance state was used as a vehicle for appropriate information. Over six months Reuben learnt to sleep well; his unconscious realised that he lived in Australia, that he was 60 years old and above all that he was safe.

The process of helping Reuben involved using hypnosis to discover what had caused his problem and educating his unconscious so it could let go of an out-of-date defence mechanism.

It is important during hypnotherapy for psychosomatic illness:

1. To explain that the illness is not the fault of the patient and that it is beyond conscious control in the same way as organic disease, thereby removing guilt.

2. To explain the mechanism of such illnesses where the mind–body connection is using the symptom for a specific purpose which may be inappropriate and out of date.

3. To teach the patient self-hypnosis so communication between the conscious and unconscious can be improved.

4. Finally, to make use of the trance state to: discover the aims of the symptom – what it is trying to do for the patient; and re-educate the unconscious as to a more up-to-date and appropriate way of dealing with the problem.

The therapy Therese received is an example of the above format.

Therese was a 40-year-old mother who had suffered from intermittent back pain for the past two years. It had begun when she strained her back lifting one of her children and had not responded to treatment.

She mentioned that when she was 12 years old she had been ice-skating and had fallen over heavily on her back. She had been terrified someone would run over her fingers with their skates.

I discussed the concept of psychosomatic pain and talked about it being beyond her control, not her fault and that she was not a malingerer. We talked about mind–body connections, how the body stores memories of past events and how hypnosis can be used to improve and update those messages. I taught Therese self-hypnosis and asked her to practise it daily so we could use the trance state to explore further.

At the following session Therese went into a trance of her own accord and I directed her to 'go into the back pain' and learn about its function. Therese remembered and relived the skating accident as if it was stored vividly in her back. She showed all the fear and anxiety that the little girl had experienced. We went over the accident again and again until she was able to relegate it to the past and resolve the emotions involved.

We then relived the experience of two years previously. I believed this had triggered her skating accident memory. She again went down in her mind to the back pain and reassured it that it no longer needed to keep muscle tension there as a protection.

Over two months' therapy and constant self-hypnosis Therese lost her back pain and was able to go to exercise classes to build up her back muscles, reduce the tension in them and be much more flexible during her daily activities.

She demonstrated how a traumatic incident in the past can remain dormant, stored in the memory for many years and then be triggered by a similar feeling causing a chronic condition.

Often psychosomatic illness has a vague, rather than specific, cause. General tension, anxiety, guilt and fear may underlie somatic symptoms. It is as though continuous energy, sent around the nervous system by a troubled mind, can cause dysfunction of the body's mechanisms.

Muscular tension from chronic fear causes pain. Bowel symptoms can result from constant worry. Anxiety may create the bronchial spasm that occurs in asthma. Guilt resulting in self-punishment can generate a variety of physical problems.

The 'Sherlock Holmes' approach to tracking down the exact cause of a symptom is often not applicable. A childhood spent with unsuitable parenting can cause great disturbance in mind–body communication; general support, understanding, relaxation and psychotherapy may be required to resolve underlying conflicts.

Often we 'blame' the symptom and curse it for the discomfort it brings. I hear comments such as: 'My stupid asthma is ruining my life' or 'This ridiculous headache is the scourge of my life.'

In my experience, having a more understanding attitude to our symptoms is much more helpful. Realising that the lungs or head are not 'responsible' for the discomfort but 'recipients' of the influence of the unconscious mind and being caring and supporting towards these parts often has a beneficial effect.

The mind–body connection plays a major role in many illnesses. Being aware of this fact, and not ashamed to accept it, is the start of a process leading to recovery.

PART 3

Specific Uses of Hypnosis

14

Pain

The strain in pain lies mainly in the brain.
Dr David Spiegel, American Psychiatrist

Those who do not feel pain seldom think it is felt.
Dr Johnson

There are two types of pain – acute and chronic. Hypnosis works well with both but is more effective in acute pain as there are not the multitude of associated difficulties that are involved with chronic pain.

Acute Pain

Hypnosis is used in cases of acute pain such as operations, trauma or accidents, where putting someone into a trance reduces sensations registered by the brain. It is relatively easy to direct someone to imagine keeping their hand in ice-cold water until it is numb at which point no pain is felt from a pin prick. Analgesia (the absence of pain) is one of the phenomena of hypnosis (see p. 74).

Hypnosis started to become widely accepted only after Dr James Esdaile performed operations in India in the mid-nineteenth century using hypnosis as the anaesthetic. In the trance state, suggestions of numbness, lack of feeling and dissociation (see pp. 66–9) are given so that the patient's mind is focused away from the painful area.

Don was a 40-year-old chef who had severe toothache, but his fear of needles was preventing him seeing a dentist. He told me that when he was a child he had a dentist who told him the needle wouldn't hurt but it did. However, the pain in his mouth was forcing him to face his fear.

We talked at length about needles, the benefits of the local anaesthetic and the discomfort caused by the injection. I explained to him I would go through the process in stages in order to help him realise it would be comfortable for him to have an injection.

When I showed him a needle and encouraged him to hold it, he looked terrified. As he began to realise he was in control he relaxed a little. Then I taught him self-hypnosis and asked him to imagine a part on the back of his right hand that was ice-cold and numb. He signalled when he had achieved that and I told him I would pinch his right hand and then the left and he was to tell me the difference.

'I didn't feel the right hand but the left hurt a little.'

'If you had the same feeling in the right hand when a needle went in would that be all right?'

He nodded.

'Would it be all right for me to put a needle in the numb part now?'

He waited a long time before slowly nodding. I inserted the needle into the skin of his right hand. Don didn't move.

'When you are ready open your eyes and look.'

He slowly opened his eyes.

'I can't believe it. Is it a trick?' he exclaimed.

'No. You were able to make that part of your hand go numb. And you can do that in the dentist's chair just as easily.'

In between sessions he practised self-hypnosis and making different parts of his body go numb. He agreed to visit his dentist and I rang him to explain what was happening and to go very slowly with Don to allow him time to go into a trance. The dentist was very co-operative and the dental procedure went smoothly.

Chronic Pain

This condition is very different from acute pain because so many different emotions appear as the pain continues. Hope is raised and dashed and the lack of control causes great concern. In order to analyse this condition I would like to describe a Pain Clinic in a teaching hospital where patients with chronic pain attend for relief. The clinic is similar to other outpatient clinics – crowded with patients; short of furniture and time. Waiting varies but is often up to two hours, and a consultation with the doctor lasts from 10 to 30 minutes.

The patients are a complete cross-section of the community. Pain is no discriminator and is the common link between all those seeking help. Chronic pain spells a history of suffering, depression, frustration, anger and fear.

The patients walk, hobble, limp, are wheeled into the clinic or brought in on trolleys. They gather in the corridors, philosophers all, wise in the knowledge of their experience

and discussing with intense looks and shaking heads the
acts of their tragedy. The stories continue: out of work five
years with a bad back; marital discord due to chronic
headaches; inability to walk due to painful hips; difficulty in
driving a car due to a stiff neck; and so on.

There is a constant attempt to understand 'why?'. There
seems to be no answer as to why the pain started or is
continuing year after year. The doctors are concerned at
their limitations to stem the flow of woeful tales that
continue to pour out at each session. They are frustrated by
their lack of knowledge or their ability to deal with this
soul-destroying problem and are eager to find a solution.

The treatments are many and varied. Some patients have
had operations to help the pain and are referred on when
the pain persists. All have been through myriad attempts to
remove the pain by their local doctors, osteopaths, chiro-
practors, herbalists or faith healers before they arrive at the
Pain Clinic.

The clinics carry out tests – X-rays, blood tests, diag-
nostic injections – to ascertain the site of the pain and what
may be causing it. It is frequently more difficult to arrive at
a precise answer than in other areas of medicine. The diag-
nostic tools are limited because the problem is subjective –
that is, the pain is only measurable by asking the patients
how they feel, rather than using a scientific instrument.
Chronic pain is a leveller. From the judge to the prisoner
all are reduced in stature by their tormentor's powers of
erosion.

How can we tackle this immense problem? There are so
many attempted solutions that there must be more than one
answer. Each form of therapy has a place, some more
helpful than others.

When the diagnosis is made and a treatable underlying

condition ruled out, the battle begins. Injections of local anaesthetic are given to block the pain pathway or cortisone injections to alter the tissue response. Success may be short-lived, long-lasting or non-existent, only time and trial can tell. Tablets and pills of all shapes, sizes and strengths are used to defeat the pain, provide relief, promote blissful sleep, wash away the day's memories. Many chronic pains are greatly helped by analgesics and the aim is to provide maximum relief with minimum side-effects. If this regime has no success, alternative therapies are used.

Acupuncture is beneficial in many cases. This time-honoured oriental therapy is increasing in popularity and success. Many people who doubted its effect are pleasantly surprised at the relief obtained after a few visits. Side-effects are minimal and the acupuncture needles are so fine that the discomfort is generally of no consequence.

Nerve stimulating machines (TENS) are small boxes strapped to an appropriate part of the body and worn under the clothes. They transmit low frequency electrical impulses to the skin in order to relieve pain. The method by which this works is related to: increasing the endorphins – naturally occurring hormones that relieve pain; intercepting pain signals from the brain; or increasing blood flow to the painful part. Many people find these very beneficial in reducing the pain to a tolerable level.

But for all those who leave the Pain Clinic smiling, there are many who return time after time, the pain still not under control. The persistence of chronic pain affects the sufferer in innumerable ways. It is a constant shadow throwing its gloom over every aspect of life, reducing enjoyment and happiness. The total range of emotions which may be released by this tormentor are anger, frustration, guilt, sadness, self-doubt and desperation. The fact that no logical reason can be given for its existence adds fuel to the emotional fire.

If you are a sufferer of chronic pain you may recognise some of these feelings. My aim will be to help you understand the pain and perhaps approach it in a slightly different way using hypnotic techniques so that you can be involved with reducing or removing it.

Firstly, I'd like to discuss attitudes towards pain and then interweave hypnosis to change negative feelings to positive ones of gaining control. I do not wish to promote hypnosis as the answer to chronic pain. I believe it plays a major role, in conjunction with other forms of therapy, or on its own.

Take Responsibility for Your Pain

You may ask, 'How do I do that? I don't know what caused it, I'm not to blame for it.' I agree – I'm not entering a moral discussion; I am saying it is your pain. Other people may try and help, but in the long run it is your problem and any way you can become involved with treating it will be to your advantage. Setting your mind to take responsibility and being prepared to spend your own time doing something for it means you are heading in the right direction.

The most common attitude is, 'Doctor, here is my pain, I don't want anything to do with it, you fix it.' In other areas of medicine this may be appropriate; for a high proportion of people with chronic pain, it is not. Learning what part you can play in understanding and reducing the pain is a difficult concept to grasp but I will point out methods of doing this using hypnosis.

The aim is to utilise the powers of the conscious and unconscious mind to rid the body of this unrelenting distress. If you consider pain as a parasite draining you of energy, the more you can learn about its habits and life-styles, the easier it will be to find a way to get rid of it.

I do not believe there is any benefit in dividing chronic pain into organic (where pathology can be demonstrated by tests and X-rays) and psychosomatic or functional pain (where no pathology of the tissues can be shown). My understanding is that pain is pain and the sufferer of chronic pain feels the same intensity of discomfort whether it is caused by the body or the mind. The treatment using hypnotic techniques may well be the same in each case. Unfortunately a stigma has become attached to psychosomatic pain as if the sufferer was to blame, had intentionally caused it and should feel guilty, as if it is his fault in some way and no one can help him.

Nothing could be further from the truth. Unfortunately, due to lack of training, some in the medical profession, unable to treat non-organic pain, label it as 'neurotic malingering' and increase the aura of guilt and blame.

The inference often is that if it is organic and tests show pathology it is acceptable; if no abnormality can be found, nothing much can be done so don't waste the doctor's time.

The Mind and Chronic Pain

All pain is felt in the mind. Whatever part of the body is affected the pain centre is in the brain and learning to use the mind to limit pain is often very helpful.

Hypnosis, learning to control some aspects of the mind, acts in many different ways to reduce pain.

Distraction

We can all forget things for a brief period of time when distracted by something exciting or enjoyable. The mind cannot concentrate on everything at once so if pain being top priority is pushed down the scale by something else it will diminish accordingly. Using self-hypnosis we can learn to use the 'forgetting part' of our mind to minimise the pain. Learning to concentrate on the comfortable parts of our body may seem difficult but it is not impossible. Going into a dream-like state and recalling happy memories will automatically provide relief from the pain. This relief may last long after the trance has finished.

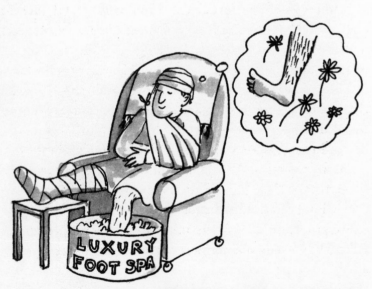

Learning to concentrate on the comfortable parts of the body may seem difficult but it's not impossible.

Helmut is an Office Manager with a very busy and hectic job. He is constantly under pressure. He had a kidney stone removed three years prior to seeing me and had constant, intense pain in a nerve involved in the operation scar. He had been in hospital on and off for the pain and the nerve had been cut, frozen, lasered and cauterised, all with no relief.

The poor man was distraught from the saga of doctor versus nerve in which he was the continual loser. When I saw him I asked him how I could help. He said, 'If only I could have a little relief each day I could cope.'

I hypnotised him and asked him to imagine a scene he'd enjoyed previously. He imagined he was alone on a lovely beach in France, the sun was hot, the water blue and the sand fine and warm under his feet. He stayed on that beach in his mind for half an hour and his face showed the appreciation of that relief as he opened his eyes.

He learnt to do self-hypnosis and for ten minutes twice a day he went to his French beach. Although he didn't develop a suntan he gained all the benefit of a brief holiday from his hectic work.

After a few weeks he noticed the pain had diminished during the rest of the day and he decided to cut his work-load and relax more. After three months the pain was negligible and he was once again able to enjoy life. Helping him to use his mind to distract his attention briefly, allowed him to gain control of the pain.

Removing negative emotions

Due to the disturbing nature of the pain or because of emotional situations involved in its causation, many negative feelings may become intertwined in the pain itself. If these can be disentangled the suffering is often remarkably relieved.

I call negative emotions those which direct the sufferer to feel worse and add a burden to the problem. Such emotions as anxiety, fear, guilt, self-punishment and conflict, all may play a role in causing or maintaining the pain.

Hypnosis is an ideal way of understanding these components and putting them into a realistic perspective. By reassessing the value of the negative component and analysing it 'in the light of day', it often disappears.

Guilt

If the pain is caused in an accident and someone else is hurt or killed, the pain may be maintained by the guilty feeling. Guilt requires punishment; what better punishment than long-term pain.

In hypnosis, reassessing the guilt, adding logic and understanding, having an imagined trial and alteration of sentence often reduce the guilt and allow the 'punishing pain' to diminish.

Mrs Johnson, a 30-year-old housewife, had always been very nervous and tense. She had been driving home one night two years previously and failed to see a child on a zebra crossing. She braked hard but knocked the child over. She thought she had killed him. In fact, he was only shaken and after a short while walked home.

The instant flash in her mind that she had killed him remained with her. For two years she had an unusual pain in her joints which remained despite investigation and treatment with umpteen tablets.

She agreed to try hypnosis only after she realised it was

her last chance. She was very dubious and fearful of 'meddling with her mind' and required her husband to sit with her at all times.

She relaxed gradually and after a few sessions was able to do self-hypnosis at home with a tape I made. During these trances she reassured her unconscious mind that she did not kill the boy and did not need the punishment she was receiving. She also learnt to relax more.

After five sessions her pain was much less; it was still present but not nearly so limiting or destructive to her life. She continued to reassure her unconscious mind and gradually she no longer needed to see me or to continue punishing herself for a crime she did not commit.

Fear

Many patients whose pain continues unexplained and untreatable develop a fear that there is an underlying condition, such as cancer, which is being missed. This fear is reinforced by the repeated efforts to prove there is no cancer. Every negative test seems to point to the fact that cancer must be present but the test is not meticulous enough. Each failed attempt to identify and remove the pain is proof that 'something' is causing it. 'The pain is real doctor, I know you don't believe me but it is destroying my life.' Any discussion seems to make matters worse and further tests seem to deepen the quicksand.

The continuous cycle of hopes raised and dashed, and therapy endlessly altered, adds to the problem. It becomes illogical – that is, out of control of the logical, conscious mind. This is where hypnosis is useful; it avoids logic and deals with the emotional aspects of the unconscious mind. The calming effect, the altered attitude, the reassuring evidence, are put to the unconscious mind to lessen the fear. Optimistic thoughts are included in the self-hypnotic routine.

Often in such cases seeking the cause of the pain takes priority over the pain itself. Talking to patients they continually ask, 'Why?' and when I say, 'Would it be all right to lose the pain and never know why it existed?' the answer is often a shake of the head. Because no one can give an answer as to why a pain persists, some of these sufferers continue on their endless quest, adding all sorts of emotional problems along the way.

A comparison between pain and a burglar alarm seems relevant. The alarm notifies us something is wrong in the house, and we take steps to investigate and use appropriate action, turning off the alarm when we are reassured that all is well. If there is a fault in the system and we leave the alarm on for days, weeks or months it serves no purpose. It will upset the household, disturb the neighbours and certainly have no effect on any intruder.

The alarm can be safely turned off or down with no detrimental effects. So it is with chronic pain; the message is no longer useful, it no longer warns us or causes us to take appropriate action. The pain can be diminished with safety, even if we do not know the cause, so long as suitable medical tests show no underlying, treatable disease.

Anxiety

Generalised anxiety from a chronic stressful condition such as pain may reinforce the situation. The hopelessness of it all, the lack of direction or understanding, all drain the energy and resources of the sufferer. Going from place to place, having test after test, treatment after treatment, spawns a downward emotional spiral. Loss of job, the humility of the dole, being dependent rather than a breadwinner, being treated as an invalid, all cause massive disruption to personality and self-esteem.

Hypnosis, by its very nature, lessens anxiety, producing a calming effect, and so may stem the flow of strength and determination 'down the drain'. Intertwined with this is the realisation that 'someone understands', 'someone is prepared to spend time with me, listen to me and acknowledge that I am not putting it all on'. The hypnotherapist often takes an understanding, supportive role in guiding people through their difficulties.

One of the problems is the non-acceptance of hypnosis as a form of therapy: 'If hypnosis can help it must be in my mind, I must be mad', and this is wrong. Many patients refuse to contemplate hypnosis as a choice on these grounds; they prefer to continue the never-ending search for a physical treatment that will take away the pain.

In a pain clinic I asked 100 consecutive patients with chronic pain the following three questions:

1. If you trusted your doctor and he recommended tablets for your pain would you take them?

2. If you trusted your doctor and he recommended an operation would you have it?

3. If you trusted your doctor and he recommended hypnosis would you let yourself be hypnotised?

I was amazed at the replies I received:

1. 100 per cent said they would take tablets.

2. 65 per cent said they would have an operation; 15 per cent said they would think about it; and 20 per cent said they would not.

3. 40 per cent said they would allow themselves to be hypnotised; 20 per cent said they would think about it; and 40 per cent said they would not.

What amazed me was that more people would accept an operation with all the pain, side-effects and dangers, than hypnosis with none of those problems. The fear of having 'their minds meddled with' was so great that even the remote possibility that their pain might be diminished was not enough stimulus to 'have a go'.

The attitude that 'it's not in the mind, doctor' also added to their negative response and this attitude is a very real, limiting factor in the general acceptance of hypnosis as a useful tool for pain relief.

Anger

Many patients are understandably angry and this may be recognised or repressed, expressed or blocked. The cause varies considerably and may be due to an initial incident where the anger was involved. As the pain continues there are multiple opportunities for creating anger but not many targets on which to vent it.

Recurring mishaps, doctors who fail in some way, misunderstandings, the pain or painful part of the body itself, the hospital, operations, etc., all may be the source of anger; but the poor patient is in no position to express anger at his potential saviour.

A young boy was knocked off his bike by a drunken driver. He received severe injuries to his leg and developed a permanent limp. Some years later he still had a lot of pain in spite of repeated attempts to control it. On the surface he appeared calm and resigned to his fate and had accepted all the pushing and waiting around which occur in chronic cases. He was also involved in legal action where the delays were interminable and he was receiving no suitable response to his questions.

After seeing him a few times it became apparent to both of us that he was understandably very angry. He was angry at the drunk who knocked him off his bike, angry at the medical profession for not curing his condition, angry at the legal profession for their delays, angry at his leg for ruining his life, angry at the pain for the discomfort it caused. I taught him ways to express his righteous anger and 'get it out' of his system. He recognised that it was acceptable to feel anger and there were some avenues where he could show this without destroying his hope of help. He wrote letters to all the people he was angry with and stated in no uncertain terms how he felt. He didn't post the letters. He made tapes about his thoughts and feelings and described in detail what he thought of the people and situations that had ensnared him. He didn't listen to the tape.

After a few weeks he felt much better; he was stemming the pent-up anger caught in his chronic pain system, and by reducing this energy he relieved the pain. He also used the relaxation and analgesia of self-hypnosis to help the overall situation.

Attitude to the painful area

After part of the body, say a limb, has been causing pain for some time, it is understandable that one would get annoyed and aggravated with it. 'If only the pain would go. Cut off my leg, I'd be happier than with this blasted pain,' are words I've often heard. It is as if the painful part is looked upon as an enemy, hour after hour, day after day, year after year, a constant reminder and cause of distress.

I believe this attitude to the limb may play a part in maintaining the pain. It is as if the affected limb is saying, 'Damn you, it wasn't my fault that you had the accident. You did it and now you're blaming me for the consequences. I'll show you, I'll pay you back.'

I'm not suggesting there is any logic to this but I have found, in many cases, that altering this attitude to one of understanding and apology may completely relieve the pain.

John is a delightful 60-year-old who came to see me in a wheelchair. His right leg had been amputated above the knee three years earlier and ever since he had suffered constant intolerable 'phantom limb' pain – pain in the limb that is no longer there. It is real and causes much distress because the painful area cannot be touched – it doesn't exist in the flesh, only in the mind.

John had been subjected to every form of treatment. He had received analgesics, sedatives, sleeping tablets, injections into the stump, operations on the nerves, injections into the nervous system, all to no avail. He came to see me in desperation with tears in his eyes, saying, 'You are my last hope, I don't know what to do if you fail too.'

I had mixed feelings at being put on a pedestal, also fearing I might not be able to help this gentle, tormented man. I discussed the various aspects of hypnosis and spent some sessions just chatting to him, understanding his fears and strengths.

He had been a successful businessman but had developed arterial disease, limiting his circulation. He had been advised to rest but, as he was concerned about financial security for his family, he continued working very hard. As time went on he developed gangrene in his foot which eventually required amputation. He was most distressed after the operation and lost his confidence; the pain and the fact that he was a one-legged man got him down. He tried to use an artificial limb but it hurt. His stump constantly jerked with the nervous tension he was under, and he felt very annoyed with the leg that had literally let him down.

After a number of sessions, I taught him relaxation and the twitching in the stump was gradually brought under control. But the pain persisted. I made hypnosis tapes for him to play, but still the pain persisted. I helped him produce analgesia in the stump but it lasted only a short while.

After three months I wasn't getting anywhere and I felt I was going to have to say to him I couldn't help his pain. Then one session, for some reason, I asked him his attitude to the stump. He described his anger, frustration and annoyance at this 'non-limb' which was causing him so much trouble.

I asked him to go into a trance and remember the times he neglected his leg. He recalled many occasions since childhood where he had injured or bruised the limb in accidents, horse-riding incidents, falls, etc. I then asked him about times he didn't treat or rest the leg when it was required. In particular he hadn't rested when advised to do so three years ago and gangrene had set in. I suggested that perhaps his leg was angry with him for all the problems he had caused it. Perhaps he should assume an apologetic attitude towards it now.

He agreed to spend time each day talking and apologising to his leg. And, wonder of wonders, the pain started to recede. It wasn't all plain sailing but from that point on we began winning the battle with the painful phantom limb. Over the next three months the pain completely disappeared. He still needed to take a mild sleeping tablet for some time to ensure a good night's sleep, but he is now able to enjoy time with his wife, children and grandchildren. He also says with a smile, 'I still pay my daily dues of respect to my old friend the "little leg".'

Muscle spasms

Pain often produces muscle spasm in the area surrounding it. A headache may be caused or maintained by tension in the neck or scalp muscles. As relaxation is part of the hypnotic experience, this may be put to great use in reducing the spasm and hence breaking the pain–spasm cycle as in the diagram below.

To demonstrate the effect of tissue tension on pain, open out your left hand and pinch some loose skin on the back, registering how painful it is. Then, holding on to the skin, slowly clench the hand and notice how the pain increases as the skin tightens. So it is with muscle spasm and by doing self-hypnosis and relaxation this muscle tension can be greatly reduced.

Reducing pain

Hypnosis can produce analgesia: using the trance state, patients can imagine part of their body going numb. This imagined numbness can produce real diminution in sensation. In the daydream-like state of a trance, patients are asked to imagine that one hand is immersed in ice-cold water. As the coldness continues, numbness develops; this numbness may be transferred to the painful area. Using thermometers to measure skin temperature it can be shown that a very marked reduction in temperature can result using this method.

Terry had chronic backache. He was unable to lift his young baby because of the pain. He had been off work for two years and was becoming depressed at being on the dole.

He was suitable for hypnosis and developed the ability to make his back numb by imagining ice on it. When he came out of the trance and moved around, the pain returned. After many visits with no lasting improvement I asked him to go into a trance, make his back numb and come out of the trance from the neck upwards. In other words, he was to leave his back in the trance but bring his head out.

Terry looked perplexed at my request but did so and was surprised that he no longer had the pain when he walked around. I asked him to go outside and walk down the street. When he returned he had the same bemused look on his face so I knew his back was 'still asleep'. He touched his toes and did many things he had not done for many months.

Pain as a Message

As with other illnesses, I believe that in many cases chronic pain may be a message which if understood leads to the pain improving. Hypnosis is an ideal state for decoding these messages, and tackling the problem this way rather than 'taking away' the pain is often successful. I would like to relate an unusual case of this kind.

Philip was a 40-year-old jeweller who had experienced joint pains for as long as he could remember. As a child, he had missed many weeks of school due to these pains, and seen numerous doctors, but no real diagnosis was made or cure effected. He had taken 'almost every pill in the book' to try and remove the pain.

Most days the pains occurred in one or more joints and he came home to rest in the middle of the day to relieve the discomfort. His family life was very happy and there was no obvious stress or emotional upset apart from the nuisance value of his continuing pain.

He agreed to use hypnosis to find out more about the pains and was a co-operative subject, easily going into a trance. I asked him to indicate when the pain had occurred the first time, as I counted back from his present age of 40.

At the age of three his mother had died. His father, a poor Australian graduate doctor, couldn't afford to keep him and he was adopted by a couple who moved to England.

When he came out of the trance he explained that he knew all this and he also knew his father was still a doctor in Australia. He had never contacted him as he did not want to cause any problems.

I tried to figure out how the pain could be a message from the time his mother died and he was adopted. Then I had a brainwave. Could it be possible that the pain was trying to help the little boy find his real father by constantly directing him to visit doctors? Illogical, but the unconscious mind often works on childish logic.

I explained my thoughts to him, how the pain was an obsolete message to find his father. He went away thinking about that and practising a relaxation technique. He was pleasantly surprised over the next two months as the pain gradually disappeared. The suffering he had experienced for 40 years was no longer necessary when he realised how out of date the message was.

Pain can be used to transmit messages which are not so dramatic as Philip's. It can represent self-punishment, attention-seeking, conflict, a message to spend more time on yourself, to relax more, to stand up for yourself, and many more. It is only by questioning under hypnosis that some of these messages can be deciphered and a course of action decided upon.

Hypnosis and going into the pain

I have found that by directing patients into the pain – that is, in the opposite direction to the one they usually choose – many aspects of the pain can be analysed. In a trance 'going into the pain and being there' helps us learn about its various components. I divide them artificially into descriptions which may be applied to the feeling. Again, this is not logical, just helpful.

I ask patients to concentrate their mind on the pain and to describe:

1. The colour of the pain.
2. The temperature.
3. Whether the muscles are tense or relaxed.
4. Whether there are associated memories stored in the pain.
5. What emotions are related to the pain.
6. Their attitude towards the pain.
7. The physical limits (outline or shape).
8. How it sounds.
9. Any message the pain may have.
10. How it feels.

Instead of running away from the pain I direct them towards it in order to dissect and understand it.

For example, a man with chronic headaches described them in reference to the above categories, as:

1. Red.
2. Hot.
3. Tense.
4. The cause of missing many outings.
5. Anger at doctors for not curing the headaches.
6. Angry at them, blaming them for a lot of problems with work and home life.
7. Like a plate pressing on my head.
8. No sound.
9. No message.
10. Like pressure.

I next asked him to make some alterations to these components using his imagination when in a trance.

1. Envisage the red changing to a relaxing blue.
2. Picture a block of ice on his head to reduce the temperature.
3. Relax the muscles.
4. Realise the memories are from the past and let them go.
5. Deal with the anger he had felt for the doctors.
6. Alter his blaming attitude to one of understanding and tolerance.
7. Envisage the plate to be smaller.
8. Imagine a soothing, relaxing sound.
9. See if any message comes to mind as you think about the pain.
10. Imagine the pressure to be lifted, lighter.

He practised this daily for ten minutes and, with much

guidance, he gradually learnt more about his headaches, what they meant to him and how to control them. After a few months, the headaches became much less frequent and less severe. One of the messages the headaches were giving him was to relax more and when he did this the message was no longer needed.

Sleep

People with constant pain sleep poorly. Sleep loss adds to the problem and lowers the pain tolerance. The night is very long if you are in pain and your partner is snoring away blissfully. Hypnosis and sleep tapes are very helpful in improving this situation (see Chapter 20).

A Final Word on Pain

All in all, chronic pain still has the upper hand. I have illustrated ways hypnosis may help. I do not suggest that it is useful in every case or that it can 'cure' chronic pain. I do maintain that it is a very helpful tool amongst all the others we have to offer and may be used in conjunction with any other therapy to alleviate pain.

It is important that you do not get the idea that all these patients lost their pain easily in a short time. There are many hurdles to overcome in order to achieve comfort. It needs an astute therapist, and a co-operative patient who has rapport with the therapist, to get the best results.

I have only mentioned 'success' stories here. Unfortunately hypnosis does not work for everyone with chronic pain. Other techniques, tablets or therapies may be required to reduce the pain to an acceptable level. Hopefully, as we learn more about hypnosis, the ratio of successes to failures will increase.

If you do have pain I suggest you try to develop the ability to use self-hypnosis and in the process learn more about your particular pain. In that way you may be able to wrest control from the relentless intruder.

15

Stress

More than any other time in history, mankind faces a crossroads. One path leads to despair and utter hopelessness. The other to total extinction. Let us pray we have the wisdom to choose correctly.

Woody Allen

Stress is a word that is becoming more and more popular in the press, in books and in medical circles. It has been quoted as the 'modern-day killer', 'the underlying cause of most diseases', 'the high cost of progress', and so on. Many volumes have been written about stress, its cause and effects. What I have to say here will be a summary of a number of thoughts and ideas to help you understand how stress may be affecting your life, and how to deal with it.

What is Stress?

The dictionary definition in relation to physical stress can also be applied to the emotions – 'a force or system of forces producing deformation or strain'. We are all under some form of strain; the only person with no stress is a dead one.

A gradation exists between creative or constructive stress and destructive or immobilising stress.

I go to bed at night and realise I haven't put out the milk bottles. I feel a minimal irritation over this, get up and put them outside the door. This is constructive stress.

I go to bed at night, realise I haven't put out the milk bottles. I develop severe anxiety at the thought of going outside; perhaps I'll be mugged. I toss and turn undecided what to do, the tension mounts, I dwell on the problem for hours, I can't sleep. This is destructive, immobilising stress as it taxes the mind and body with no resolution.

Numerous variations on this theme occur in most people's lives. The physical reaction to stress is called a 'flight or fight' reaction. This means that chemicals and hormones are produced in the body either to fight or run away from the

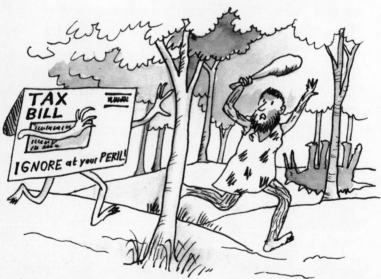

Due to the demise of the dinosaur our modern day stressful situations are not solved by the foot or club method.

stressful situation. These reactions began millions of years ago as a means of survival. Prehistoric animals without this system, calmly grazing while a predator approached, would not have lived long enough to worry about putting out the milk bottles.

As man evolved, he developed this fight or flight response to stress – a constructive reaction to deal with a hungry dinosaur – and either used his club or his feet to advantage. Due to the demise of the dinosaur our modern-day stressful situations are not solved by the foot or club method. Vastly different and more subtle ways are needed to subdue it.

So the internal reactions which help fight or flight, that is, increased blood pressure, pulse rate, breathing, sweating and muscular tension, have no outlet in modern society. But this process places an immense long-term strain on the body and the mind.

In fact this 'stress syndrome', as it is called, feeds upon itself. The more stressed we become the more tense, anxious and worried we are, which in itself produces stress. So a vicious (and that is a very appropriate word) cycle is set up, leading, in many cases, to physical or emotional symptoms.

The whole subject of stress can be divided into two components:

1. **The stressor**, that which causes stress and this could be either: *external* – some event or situation that is causing stress; or *internal* – attitudes or emotions that lead to stress (anxiety, guilt, low self-esteem, self-blame, fear, etc.).

2. **Our reaction to the stressor** – how we deal with it, how our body responds, what emotions are involved.

External stressors

These are events that produce stress and range from a stubbed toe to a traffic jam. In the times of the caveman the stressor was a predator and a normal resting state was maintained after the predator was dispatched. In today's society the predator (the bank manager or tax inspector) is constantly with us, so no return to the resting state occurs.

Our bodies have not changed with the times and our protective stress reaction deals with the stressor using out-of-date weapons. In fact it's as if the weapons are so rusty they explode in our hands when fired at the enemy.

When we are caught in a traffic jam and feel the adrenaline flow in readiness, it is of no use to fight or fly: we are hemmed in and the taxi driver in front is six foot six and 18 stone. So, understandably, we sit fuming in the car thinking of all the problems which will ensue, while the stress reaction causes all sorts of havoc in our body.

There are innumerable external events that trigger off a stress reaction. They are not universal; some people become anxious about an aeroplane flight, others about giving a speech. The common factor is the stress response to an external stimulus.

Internal stressors

These stimuli come from inside, from our minds. Because of certain attitudes and emotions we become stressed in response to our thoughts. Chronic worries can create stress from almost any situation.

- 'I've noticed a spot on my forehead, what if it is cancer?'
- 'My friend is coming for supper, what if the meal doesn't turn out correctly?'

- 'I'm never going to get my work done, life is just too much for me.'

There are a variety of different groups of people who bring these stresses upon themselves – people who are worriers, anxious, perfectionists, jealous, frightened, insecure, shy – all create internal stressors by their attitudes.

As the world is a changing place, those who place great emphasis on control have a difficult time; people who fear change are constantly battling with the natural changes that take place around them. Stress reactions cover the spectrum of mental and physical disorders: headaches, hypertension, ulcers, heart attacks, bowel disorders, pain, skin conditions, irritability, pre-menstrual tension, asthma, insomnia, 'nervous breakdown', to name a few.

Many doctors believe our immune system efficiency is reduced by stress. This may be the underlying cause of infections and even cancer, as the body's defence mechanisms are depleted by the constant fight against the dinosaurs of the past. It would be hard for me to overestimate the problems stress may cause. Hypnosis and relaxation are very successful ways of dealing with stress. It is important for you to realise first that you are under stress; then I will explain ways to reduce this to a safer level.

How Do You Know if Stress is Affecting You?

There are a multitude of signs, some of which are obvious, and others which require a trained eye to detect.

Let us take an imaginary morning in the life of John Smith, insurance salesman, average man with a wife, two kids, house mortgaged, car on hire purchase.

At 7 a.m. the alarm bell rings, starting him off in an irritated mood. It is raining. His wife gives him a peck on the cheek and gets to the bathroom first. He looks at the clock and thinks, 'I'm going to be late', and lights up the first fag of the day.

His wife takes longer in the bathroom than he expects, he goes downstairs, lets the dog out, and picks up the mail. All the letters have windows – bills for the car and house: electricity, telephone, gas, plumber, etc.

The kids are screaming because they can't find their socks. The dog is jumping all over the bed with muddy paws. When he gets to the bathroom he looks in the mirror through the smoke haze and doesn't like (or even recognise) what he sees. He lathers his face for a shave, turns on the tap, the water runs cold. His wife's shower has used all the hot water.

And so it goes on. Is it not understandable that our body, equipped to deal with brontosauruses, has trouble with cold shaving water? Stressors are everywhere. Hidden in the cupboard is a shoelace about to break, keys hide themselves under cushions, shirts develop a stain in the wrong place at the wrong time, and so on.

In those situations, we do not need a portable adrenaline meter to know we are under stress, the glance in the mirror tells us that. But there are many long-term events causing stress which we do not recognise. These events may be in the past, but the memory in the back of our minds still creates the stress reaction of panic, nervous tension, irritability, etc.

In order to detect if stress is affecting you, let's look at the various systems of the body and mind. What we are looking for are signs of stress that are not being dealt with satisfactorily.

1. *The skin and mouth* Excess sweating, skin rashes, itching, blushing, psoriasis, eczema, boils, dermatitis, hair loss, worry wrinkles from constant frowning, nail-biting, recurrent skin infections, teeth grinding, aching jaws, recurrent throat infections, mouth ulcers.

2. *The muscles* Increased muscle tightness, tension or tremors. These are commonly found in the neck or scalp, jaws, shoulders, back muscles, abdomen, clenched fists. Often this constant tension causes pain in the area.

3. *The heart and blood vessels* Palpitations, angina, heart attacks, high blood pressure, chest pains.

4. *Gastrointestinal system* Recurrent diarrhoea or constipation, bowel cramps, indigestion or peptic ulcers, abdominal pains, increased wind, irritable bowel syndrome.

5. *The nervous system* Nerves 'on edge', headaches, insomnia, depression, anxiety, uncontrolled temper, wide mood swings, memory loss, nervous habits, chronic tiredness, 'uptight', 'not able to cope', etc.

6. *Weight* Our weight may be a useful indication of how we cope with stressful situations. Being either overweight or underweight may be a sign that stressors are being dealt with by our eating pattern. Eating, like smoking, is one not-so-successful way of dealing with stress.

7. *Reproductive system* Pregnancy and delivery are often very stressful situations. Pre-menstrual tension, difficulty with intercourse either from the male or female side such as, painful intercourse, premature ejaculation and failure of

erection, are some of the psycho-sexual disorders, as well as reduced libido that result from strain.

You may feel I have gone 'overboard' in my list, but I can assure you I have not. I am not saying every condition mentioned is always due to stress, but stress plays a major role in many such cases.

What Can We Do to Diminish the Stress Response?

Now that you have some idea what stress is and how it may be caused, let us move to the important part of the chapter – how you can reduce the punishment your body is receiving.

There are four levels at which you can reinforce your weapons in the battle. You may choose to use one or all of these tactics.

1. Dealing with the stressor

If John's stress level rises to a fever pitch when his wife stays too long in the bathroom he could:

1. talk to her about it then or later,
2. make sure he gets to the bathroom first,
3. occupy his mind with something else such as reading the paper.

With many stressful situations there are practical alternatives to the way we handle them. I won't enumerate them but I'm sure you can think of alternative ways of behaviour (especially when not actually involved in the situation) which would be more suitable next time.

2. Altering the internal 'self-talk'

We constantly talk to ourselves in our minds. This 'self-talk' may be negative and magnify the problems we face and the associated tension. It may be painting a disastrous picture which is far from the truth.

'If she stays there much longer my breakfast will be cold, I'll miss the train and I'll have to wait 20 minutes, the next train will probably be crowded, I won't get a seat, the driver may go to sleep, the train will be derailed, we'll all be killed. All because she stays in the bloody shower all morning.'

This sort of self-talk is not very helpful. Perhaps an alternative, more appropriate, internal dialogue may be suitable: 'She's got a long day ahead with the kids and her job, and her mother's ill. I'll let her enjoy the hot water a little longer, in fact I'll slip down and get her some tea and toast when she eventually decides to come out of the bloody shower.' (See also Chapter 5 for general benefits of improving self-talk).

3. Relaxing the body

This is a very important and practical way you can reduce the stress level in your system (see also pp. 62–3). I will take you through a ten-minute relaxation exercise which I feel is 'life-saving' in many situations. Doing this exercise daily or twice daily may seem a real chore, but being off work for three months following a heart attack isn't much fun either.

Allocate a time and place to do this exercise on a daily basis. Don't find the time, make it. You should not be disturbed by the telephone, wife, kids, dog, etc. If necessary hang a sign on the door: 'Survival time, interruption may cause death'. Make sure you have no need to go to the toilet. If you like play calming music in the background.

- Sit in a comfortable chair or lie down on the bed, couch or floor. Ensure the temperature is suitable.

- When you feel comfortable concentrate on your breathing, close your eyes if it makes you feel more relaxed. Allow your breathing to become slow, not forced, more in your abdomen than your chest. At each breath out imagine you are breathing some tightness or tension out of your body.

- Concentrate on a part of your body and breathe the tension out of it. Notice the muscles becoming more relaxed as you do so.

- After a few minutes, starting at your toes and working your way up, slowly contract then relax each part of your body. I will name them in order:

Toes:	Screw up your toes, feel the tightness, then let them go. Notice the difference.
Ankles:	Pull your feet towards your head so you feel tightness in the ankles. Let go.
Calf muscles:	Tighten then relax.
Thigh muscles:	Tighten then relax.
Abdominal muscles:	Tighten then relax.
Clench fists:	Then relax them – imagine squeezing any irritating thoughts or feelings out of your body.

Bend elbows up:	Then relax them.
Shrug shoulders:	Then relax them.
Clench teeth:	Then relax and let the jaw drop open a little.
Screw up eyelids:	Then relax.
Raise eyebrows:	Then relax.
Tense neck muscles:	Then relax.

- Take a deep breath in, then slowly let it out and feel the relaxation all over your body.

- Remain in that state for a few minutes. Check that all your body is relaxed. If some part is still tense, concentrate on reducing that tension.

- After ten minutes, gradually open your eyes and slowly get up and get on with your daily life.

During the day your body may be giving you signs that stress is building up and you can help that situation by altering the body's response. If you notice your breathing is more rapid, slow it down. If your muscles are tense – jaw tight, hands clenched – loosen them. If you are assuming a tense position with neck stiff, shoulders hunched – relax them. If you notice your voice is louder, higher pitched or more rapid – slow it down.

Hyperventilation
This term is used to describe overbreathing. Many people breathe too rapidly or too deeply for their body's require-ments. This produces a decrease in carbon dioxide in the blood and many symptoms may result from this.

Learning to breathe correctly at a suitable rate, using the diaphragm rather than the chest, can make dramatic changes to how you feel. Altering an incorrect breathing pattern may transform someone from a 'nervous wreck' to a competent, relaxed person. This requires some instruction from a qualified physiotherapist as hyperventilation is often a long-standing habit.

In order to tell if you are a hyperventilator, place one hand on your chest and the other on your abdomen. Breathe normally and notice if the upper or lower hand is moving. If it is the upper hand you are breathing incorrectly and this may be an underlying cause of unexplained symptoms. If your lower hand is moving and the upper hand is still, then you are using your diaphragm, which is the correct organ for breathing at rest. The chest is used for extra oxygen as in the fight or flight response.

4. Relaxing the mind

As the mind is composed of both conscious and unconscious parts it may be that you are aware (conscious) of what is causing stress or you may have no idea (unconscious) why you feel the way that you do.

The brain is made up of millions of neurones all interconnecting in an amazingly complicated way, so that every second thousands of messages are circulating in the brain both in the conscious and unconscious parts. Some of these messages may cause negative feelings of fear, anxiety, etc, so that using a method to relax the mind diminishes the messages and hence the feelings.

Humans and animals have a natural way to relax the mind – ultradian rhythm (see p. 16) – which is often overruled by the pressure of daily life. It is therefore important that we instil a routine to put back this rhythm and restore balance to the overworked neurones by relaxing them on a regular basis. Failure to do so can lead to stress exhaustion, burn-out or ME – myalgic encephalomyelitis – a condition of tiredness that requires long periods of rest to resolve.

I will now describe one method of relaxing the mind called visualisation and which I referred to on page 65. Try this after the body relaxation described earlier.

- Let us assume you have achieved relaxation in your muscles and are sitting or lying comfortably. Think of a scene you find most relaxing. This may be something you have actually experienced, seen on TV or at the cinema, or imaginary. Let me suggest walking on an isolated beach.

- Imagine yourself on holiday. You are strolling (or lying) on a lovely beach. You are all alone (or with someone you like). You feel free, secluded, yourself. The sun is shining, the sky is blue, the warmth filters right through you.

- You notice the colour of the sea, the gentle breeze; you can even smell the salt. The sound of seagulls can be heard and time is non-existent. The soft sand feels so good under your bare feet, the gentle lap of the waves on the shore makes you feel sleepy.

- You decide to lie in the warm sand, perhaps let it run through your fingers. You feel dreamy and dozy and have a wonderful appreciation of having nothing to do but just *be* there. Let your mind wander in a really passive way. Allow any thoughts of 'the other world' to pass through, don't try to stop them. Don't try at all.

- Permit yourself to be a 'receiver' of any messages from the mind or body. Let the comfort of it all flow right through you. As if energy is being restored, tension draining away into the sand.

- Just *be* there. Nothing matters, nothing to do. Allow the sounds of the scene to be a part of the relaxation; perhaps view 'the other world' from this safe distance, allowing things to settle into perspective.

- Perhaps allow some thoughts, some decisions, some commitments for an altered attitude when you 'return' there.

- Be aware of how calm, how serene, how tranquil you feel. Store that feeling for future use. Remain in that state as long as you wish.

- When you are ready gradually let yourself 'come out' of that relaxed state. You may feel refreshed as if you have had a swim in that blue water, perhaps noticing you have more energy.

Get into a routine of doing this, not when you are tired at the end of the day and in bed about to go to sleep – although it would be helpful if you have sleep problems – but first thing in the morning or at lunch time to restore your mind's capacity for dealing with stress.

Here is another example of this form of visual imagery for self-hypnosis, using a different scene:

- Stare at a specific point in front of you. Continue to look at it as if your beam of vision is connecting your eyes to that point.

- Keep your eyes open until the eyelids feel heavy and want to close. Let your mind wander, your breathing become slow and calm, your muscles relax.

- When your eyelids become heavy and it is a strain to

keep them open, allow them to close lowly, breathing out at the same time.

- Just enjoy doing nothing for a minute or so, being aware of any of your thoughts, your body, your breathing. Don't try and do anything, whatever happens is all right.

- Imagine you are at the top of some stairs. Ten stairs in all. Slowly, in your own time, count from one to ten going down one step, and matching your breathing, with each number. Maybe you'll have a picture or a feeling of the stairs.

- At the bottom of the stairs is a garden. A very special garden of your own choice. You go into the garden. You feel really good in this garden, nothing to worry you there. You stroll around the garden feeling more and more at peace, more and more tranquil, more and more your real self, all in your own time, little by little.

- You allow the world at the top of the stairs to drift away. Passively strolling around the garden, time is irrelevant; you notice the flowers, shrubs, trees. Feel the cushion-like grass under your feet, the fresh air scented with flowers, the colours of leaves and the blue sky.

- After a while you sit on a garden seat and let all the surroundings engulf you. Be there absorbing the sounds of the birds, the rustle of the leaves, the peace. Notice the warmth of the sun, the pattern of dappled light and feel the peace, serenity and calmness filtering through you.

- You may talk to yourself, give yourself advice about activities in the life at the top of the stairs. Realise the benefit that this tranquillity will have on counteracting the stress. Store the feeling for future use. Perhaps the picture or the sound or feeling of that place will come to mind at a future time.

- Notice how your body feels. Perhaps it's warm and heavy, or peaceful and floating. Notice how you don't want to move, to think, to do anything.

- Begin to learn from the plants, insects and trees around you. Notice how different they all are, yet they fit into a group, a society. The colour of each blade of grass is a slightly different shade of green; each is unique, yet fits into the overall pattern of the lawn.

- Allow the conscious, critical, controlling part of your mind to float away. It has no role in this garden. This is a passive garden which allows the back of the mind to drift into view.

- Remain there for however long you feel comfortable, take your time. When you are ready to come out of that scene, come slowly up the stairs counting from ten to one, one number for each stair on each inspiration.

- Allow a little time to enjoy the experience, whatever it was.

Each time you do this you may find it becomes easier, deeper, less under conscious control. I doubt if you will feel any change the first few times, but as you become familiar with the routine you will notice yourself gradually 'letting go'. It's as if you are exploring unknown territory: as you discover little things you will feel more secure and able to progress, and you will proceed further and further into the trance state at your own pace. Your ability to relax will increase and the tension and anxiety will diminish.

You may feel it will help to read what I have written out loud and tape-record it; listening to your voice or someone else's voice saying the words will enable you to let them passively float through your mind. I often use a tape of birdsong or waves as soothing background noise.

Performance Stress

In some areas of life when we are called upon to perform, the nervous tension involved minimises our performance. After-dinner speaking, exams, cocktail parties, driving tests, competitions, meeting strangers and many other situations, are so stressful to some people that they avoid them or 'make a mess of them'.

Using self-hypnosis to have a 'dress rehearsal' of the event and to be your own 'coach or director' will provide a means of coping with the situation in a more relaxed way.

Imagine you have had some driving lessons. Your instructor thinks you are competent and ready to take the test. You have heard so many stories of failure that you dread the day of the test and you develop panic feelings just at the thought of it.

- Allow yourself 20 minutes on your own each day.

- Do the physical relaxation mentioned earlier (pp. 172–4).

- When you are relaxed imagine setting out for the test. If you feel nervous thinking about it wait until you have calmed down before proceeding.

- Get a picture in your mind of how it will be with the instructor driving you to the test site. Let your breathing relax you.

- Imagine the examiner greeting you and asking you to lead him to your car. Remain calm and keep telling yourself you will be all right. Repeat your instructor's words of encouragement. Ignore the negative messages which may be spinning around in the back of your mind.

- Go through the test routine in your mind. Calm, comfortable and confident. It is only a test route not a war; at worst you will repeat it and learn from the experience. Correct any negative, tense-making thoughts or feelings. Go through the whole test course and then walk back with the examiner and receive his congratulations at having passed.

- Stay with that feeling for a little while and give yourself a 'pep talk' about how nice it will be when it is all over.

- Allow your eyes to open and keep any positive, confident feelings that remain.

- Do this every day and again on the morning of the test.

Similarly with exam nerves: for some weeks before, have a 're-run' of the exam in a relaxed state, and perhaps spend five minutes at the start of the exam in a relaxed state after reading the paper. This will help the knowledge held in the unconscious to filter through to the conscious mind. A recent Mastermind winner stated he used self-hypnosis before and during the competition.

Many great sportsmen have used hypnosis before and during their events too. This allows the restrictive nervous tension to be diminished. Golfers, tennis players, snooker players, all perform better if their muscles are able to move unhindered by spasms created by tension.

Panic States

In these situations the person feels a panic coming on for no apparent reason. He feels well, then gets an ominous feeling that an attack is about to occur. His pulse races, his breathing increases, he goes pale and sweaty, and has the 'indescribable feeling he is going to die'. This may last seconds or minutes and sometimes longer. The cause is most likely an unconscious memory flooding the conscious mind due to a thought or trivial incident that triggers the recall. The fear of it recurring often plays a role.

Hypnosis is a very useful technique to cure panic attacks. Learning how they first started – what triggered them off – is a good beginning. Your state of mind at the time, for instance whether you were overworked or had just ended a relationship, is a factor that may be relevant.

The treatment of panic attacks is *prevention*. They are like an explosion. It is better to put water on the fuse than try to contain the gunpowder once it has ignited. Learning self-hypnosis, and realising that you can calm yourself and achieve peace and tranquillity, builds confidence in your ability to prevent panic attacks. Slowing down is also helpful especially if you are someone who races constantly with no time for yourself.

One technique is to use self-hypnosis to achieve a deeply relaxed state and then desensitise yourself by imagining a film of the panic attack sequence while maintaining a relaxed state. Once the emotions of fear or anxiety start then stop the film and focus on rebuilding the relaxed feeling. When you are relaxed again start the film of the situation that triggers the panic.

For example, if you have panicked on the tube and are avoiding that method of travel in case it happens again, imagine the scene of preparing to go to the tube and maintain a relaxed feeling. Continue to imagine getting on to the tube until the anxiety starts. Stop the film and wait until you have calmed down before starting the film again.

Do not hurry this process; take as long as you need to proceed through the film until you have completed the journey. You may need several days to complete the journey taking half an hour a day to do the exercise. It is important that you are deeply relaxed when you do this exercise as this will then influence the deeper levels of the mind.

Stress has such a variety of ways of influencing our emotions, attitudes and behaviour. Hypnosis is one of the major ways of dealing with such a destructive condition.

16

Obesity

We live on one-third of the food we eat. Doctors and diet organisations live on the other two-thirds.

If life is a journey, obesity is the excess luggage which spoils the trip.

Brian Roet

If there is any part of our life for which we cannot delegate responsibility to other people it is for our weight. It is your hand that puts the food into your mouth. In life's other problems we find reasons outside ourselves which we can use as excuses. With weight, unfortunately, it is up to you to be in control. Yet of all the conditions we have, there are more excuses for being overweight than any other I know.

- 'I only drink twelve pints of beer a day – that won't put on weight, will it?'
- 'It's my glands, doctor.'
- 'I only have to look at food and I put on weight.'
- 'It's all the hassle of work that makes me put on weight.'
- 'It's my husband's fault; whenever he nags I binge.'
- 'The problem is I'm retaining too much fluid.'
- 'I've got big bones.'

And so it goes on, time after time; people allocate

responsibility to something or someone other than the hand that feeds them.

Obesity is a very difficult condition to cure. The profusion of diets, books, clubs, theories demonstrate that we don't have the answer. I don't have the answer either, but perhaps I can help you understand the problem a little better which may be useful in teaching you how to control your weight.

Let's start at the beginning. A baby is born with a need for milk to survive, and a metabolism to digest the milk and convert it into energy and protein for building tissues. The amount required will vary for each individual – this is an important fact to grasp.

The mother and the doctors don't know exactly how much that baby requires but they have a good approximation from experience. The only way the baby can let anyone know it needs more milk is by crying. The problem is that it may cry for other reasons, but, as we don't know what they are, we generally give milk to deal with the crying.

In time the baby may enjoy the attention associated with feeding and therefore drink when it is not necessary. Let us assume that at birth a baby has a mechanism which could be represented as:

Body needs food ⟶ hunger ⟶ crying ⟶ food
                                                               ⟱
Stop eating ◄–removal of hunger ◄–appetite control centre

After being digested, the food travels to the brain via the bloodstream. In the brain there is a small area called the appetite control centre (or satiety centre) where the food eaten is registered. It is important to realise that there is some delay between eating and registering what has been eaten.

This mechanism, which tells us when we have had enough food, is very delicately balanced. As we grow and mother dictates what we eat and when, it is constantly overridden. Instead of the child knowing and directing when he should eat, time and social factors dictate the feeding schedule so innate control is taken over. When he is not hungry and leaves some food, the child is told not to waste it but to finish what is on the plate. Meal times often develop into 'battlegrounds' where food is the ammunition for both sides rather than nourishment for the body.

So as adults we may have lost the ability or willpower to eat when required and stop when we have had enough. The perfect balance of this device is seen in wild animals: they eat when hungry and stop – leaving part of the carcass if they are carnivorous – when they have had enough. That is why we don't see fat animals, except those where humans have been involved in their feeding.

One of the main aims of weight control is to remove the layers of miscontrol which have superseded the one nature provided, and to get back to our natural individual mechanisms for starting and stopping eating.

As the baby grows the value of food is represented in many different ways. It is a link with the mother – with survival. From the mother's side it is a sign of love: she gives food, gives herself, gives love. And so food takes on a different perspective from the original need for survival, to supply the body with nourishment and build growing bodies.

Food becomes a handy convenience to deal with many aspects of life. It is handy because it is available in many forms, varieties, tastes and it is convenient because it is easily acquired, readily accessible and acceptable as the 'currency' of the culture.

- 'Poor dear, you've fallen over, have a sweetie and it won't hurt so much.'
- 'You have a cold. Have something to eat and you'll get better quickly.'
- 'You are feeling low, here, have a piece of cake, that will brighten you up.'
- 'You look tired – here, have a good cup of soup and you'll have more energy.'
- 'I'm so sad your boyfriend didn't turn up. Never mind, come and have a cup of tea and a biscuit and you'll soon forget about him.'

And so it goes on, food forever satisfying needs which are not fulfilled in other areas: food the comforter, food the pacifier, food the healer, food the carrier of love. In the back of the mind a tape is switched on: 'Food will make *it* better', 'it' covering the spectrum of negative emotions we go through during our growing years.

The fact is food does NOT make 'it' better. With over-weight people food makes it *worse* because as well as not solving the problem it adds another. Whenever things go wrong, instead of seeking a solution to the problem or an acceptance of it, the refrigerator is consulted as having the answer to all things. Self-hypnosis can be used to change the tape to 'food will not make it better'.

As the person grows and becomes overweight, the excess fat becomes involved in their lifestyle. They learn to use it for comfort, to hide behind, to punish them-selves, to gain attention, to punish others, as an excuse for failure, and so it becomes part of their way of dealing with life. As the years pass, a pattern is formed. On the one hand desperate attempts are made to lose weight – diets, calorie counting, etc. – and on the other hand there

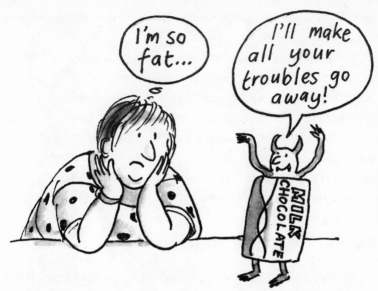

In the back of the mind a tape is switched on: 'Food will make it better.'

is a fear of losing weight because it provides such a resource to deal with problems.

Health Aspects of Obesity

As well as the psychological effects of being overweight, there are many physical problems caused or exacerbated by excess fat. The harmful symptoms are related to how much overweight people are; the more fat the greater the problem.

Statisticians, realising these harmful effects, have determined a range of normal values depending on age, sex and height and as a result insurance policies are 'loaded' if the client is overweight. Problems occur when the weight is outside this range, but the worry of being a few kilogrammes (or pounds) over probably causes more trouble than does the actual weight.

In order to simplify the medical hazards, I have listed them according to the bodily systems affected. To appreciate the body's point of view I suggest, when next in a supermarket, you count the number of bags of sugar equivalent to your excess weight. Hold the sugar and walk around with it for two minutes (if the store detective accosts you tell him are under doctor's orders) and appreciate what your body is carrying around all day.

The cardiovascular system

If you imagine a second-hand car driving around with 50 bricks on the roof, you may get an idea of the strain excess fat puts on the heart and blood vessels. The car engine is forced to perform excessively and so wear and tear on all parts is increased.

So it is with the heart; it needs to pump blood for one-and-a-half bodies when it was not constructed to do so. The strain involved in increasing the work of the heart, which beats approximately 100,000 times a day, is shown in angina, heart attacks and palpitations. If you are 6kg (14lb) overweight, hold the same amount of sugar and squat down and stand up 20 times. Then put the sugar down, do the same thing and notice the difference. Your poor heart is doing that 100,000 times a day, 365 days a year, so it's no wonder that in many cases it gives up. How would you feel towards the person who forced you to carry that sugar with you wherever you go? Perhaps that is how the heart feels towards its overweight boss.

High blood pressure is helped dramatically in most cases by losing excess weight. It is the first thing cardiologists advise before using chemical therapy. The complications of high blood pressure are strokes (cerebral haemorrhage) or heart attacks.

Respiratory system

The diaphragm moving up and down is responsible for breathing at rest. A pot belly restricts this movement and limits the breathing capacity. A common reason for seeking help for obesity is shortness of breath. 'I didn't realise what my fat was doing to me until I tried to run for a bus and puffed like an asthmatic Pekinese', or 'I walked up some stairs and I couldn't speak for five minutes I was so out of breath.' It is such a pleasure to see these people, after they have lost weight, come running up the stairs, beaming, to prove their fitness.

People with chest diseases – emphysema, bronchitis, asthma – and chronic smokers, are much more limited if they are overweight. The extra weight may be the straw that breaks the camel's back and causes death from respiratory failure.

The joints

The joints of the spine, hip, knee and ankle all bear the brunt of the extra weight. Damage to the cartilage of the joint and increased 'wear and tear' all result from the heavier load they carry. Experiments testing the internal pressure in the hip joint showed that, for every 6kg (14lb) overweight, the joint had an increased load of twice that amount due to the concentration of internal forces. Hence every 500g (1lb) lost results in a sigh of relief from the joint equal to 1kg (2lb) – that's two to one, which are good odds for any gambler.

Operations

Surgery brings the possibility of increased complications to the obese patient. For the doctor, it is more difficult to diagnose some conditions if a thick layer of fat is between the palpating hand and the diseased organ. This is especially so in abdominal or gynaecological conditions. As breathing is restricted, anaesthetic problems and risks are increased both during the operation and post operatively. The surgeon operating has practical difficulties because of the yellow fat limiting his access. Wound healing is impaired, recovery time is prolonged and surgical complications are more likely. The poor nurse in the ward who has to supervise post-operative recovery has an increased chance of injuring her back lifting and turning fat patients. So you can see how harmful being overweight is, not only to the owner of all that reserve fat, but also to those involved in their care.

As time goes by and the dislike of the extra fat becomes more intense – especially when the warm weather arrives – other feelings join the pattern. A dislike of oneself, a loss of confidence, a feeling of inferiority, all add impetus to the pathway which ends up at the refrigerator.

Other people try to help – friends, husbands, partners, but this has the reverse effect. Criticism is met with anger and food, no comment is taken as not caring, praise is taken as sarcasm, and so further eating occurs whatever attitude is adopted. It is a pattern which continues to repeat itself.

I would like to list some of the characteristics of the chronically obese person seeking medical help for the problem. These are naturally not specific for any one person but apply to the vast majority of overweight people I have seen. I hope there are no moral judgements involved in the attitude towards obesity. In my opinion it is a condition which causes an immense amount of suffering and pain and is badly understood by the medical profession and all those who have not been overweight.

- They will have been overweight for some years.
- Their weight problem started either when they were quite young, after the birth of a child or after severe emotional strain.
- Either one or both parents were overweight.
- Their mother thought or talked a lot about food and insisted they eat everything on the plate. 'Think of the poor children in India' was a common phrase at dinner time when food was left.
- They have tried many diets and weight reduction programmes.
- They feel depressed and lack confidence due to excess weight.
- Trying on clothes that once fitted, or buying new clothes which are a size larger than the previous ones, are often reasons to seek help.
- They feel people don't understand their problem, their partner is no help, and whatever they say makes things worse.
- Their visits to doctors are generally of no help and they are told it is their problem and they should eat less.
- They try to please people and be liked. They don't want to argue and have difficulty standing up for their rights.
- They don't do enough exercise and regard their over-weight body as 'the enemy'.
- They eat because they are fed up, bored, tired, depressed, anxious, lonely or upset.
- They weigh themselves constantly and talk about

weight, diets and the latest fads whenever the opportunity arises.
- They buy food with the excuse that it's for the children but eat it themselves.
- They would do anything to lose weight and feel better.
- They know more about calories and diets than the doctor they visit.
- Phrases using 'eating words' are part of their vocabulary – 'I'm fed up', 'With all my worries I've got such a lot on my plate', 'I can't get my teeth into the problem'.

So you can see weight is not an isolated problem but ties in a multitude of difficulties and deficiencies. Sometimes there is an underlying guilt feeling related to childhood experiences; perhaps a sexual misadventure brings about the mistaken belief that punishment is necessary. This punishment continues long after the incident is forgotten.

Guilt is one cause of obesity. Comfort eating is another. 'Things are lousy so I can at least comfort myself by eating.' This starts in childhood and becomes an unrecognised pattern when adulthood is reached, a habit ingrained. If you must have comfort, buying small presents (not food) for yourself, may provide the desired comfort without the price of weight.

Difficulty in being assertive can be a cause of obesity. If speaking your mind is a frightening experience then eating and being fat may provide an alternative.

Society's insistence that 'being slim is being successful' implies that anyone overweight is abnormal, an inferior citizen. This is an artificial criterion of how we should look, and attempting to fit into this concept may cause more worry than benefit.

Sometimes in a relationship the extra weight has multiple

functions. It is a focal point for tensions and arguments. It is an avenue for excuses. If the relationship is breaking down but the female partner fears leaving, then obesity may be used as an excuse for not leaving: 'If I was slimmer, I would leave and find another man, but as I'm fat no one else would have me, so I'd better stay.' It may be used to embarrass and punish the partner, part of whose belief is: 'He should like me as I am. I'm not going to lose weight just because he likes me when I'm slim.'

There are many incorrect lessons which we learn in childhood about eating which cause a lot of problems.

- 'You must have three good meals a day.'
- 'You must finish what is on the plate.'
- 'You must not eat before bedtime.'

These are incorrect because they are not based on fact but on habit. There is no evidence that we need three meals a day. This arrangement has come about for convenience to the household. If we base our eating pattern on the fact that 'food is for the body not the mind', then it is obvious that an overweight person's body does not need three meals a day. In fact more frequent, small amounts of food taken during the day are digested more easily than three large meals.

There is no reason to finish what is on the plate apart from good manners. If the body requires only half a meal it makes sense to eat only that amount. If the body doesn't require any food it seems reasonable to refuse food and enjoy the company and conversation of the dinner table.

The food will still be digested if you eat before bedtime just as it is at any other time. It may be preferable to exercise after eating but it is certainly not harmful if you don't.

There is often a grave misconception about why people

eat. Many people do so because it is the time of day to eat, or someone else is eating, or they have a feeling they label as 'hunger', which may be anything from anxiety to indigestion.

So now you may begin to understand the enormity (no pun intended) of the problem. So many factors are involved, it's no wonder that the weight-reduction industry is as lucrative as it is.

I offer no guarantees of success, but I suggest if you follow my advice you will have a much better chance of losing weight and staying slimmer. The basic aim is to eat the correct amount of food *for your body* and to *stop when you have had enough*. It is important to have suitable exercise and other ways of dealing with the stresses of life.

I am going to list the factors involved and the changes you may need to make. Obviously many of the things I mention will not apply to you, but if you have a weight problem the only way you can deal with it is by making a change in some aspect of your life. If you are not prepared to make any changes, learning to accept your obesity may be the choice for you.

1. Diets are seldom successful. A diet implies a temporary change of eating pattern with associated weight loss, followed by returning to the original pattern and accompanying weight gain.
2. Eating pattern. Examine why you eat and how you eat, what you eat.

Why You Eat

I would like you to consider yourself as a mind and a body. If you are overweight your body only needs minimal external nourishment. Your calorific requirements can be met by your body digesting or burning up the excess weight. Most people eat for the needs of their mind and not their body. Whenever you put something to your lips ask yourself, 'Does my body need this?' If the answer is 'no', don't eat it. You will say, 'But I'm always hungry.' Hunger is a feeling provided by nature to prevent you dying of starvation. What you are feeling is a habit or false hunger, because you have been eating excessively for so long.

This habit hunger may be pain, discomfort or rumbling but it is not hunger. It is not the message to eat. It may be a message about anger, loneliness, boredom, tension, none of which are resolved by food. You may have been mis-interpreting this message from your body for ages. Your appetite control centre hasn't worked properly for years and is not letting you know when you have had enough. Its wishes have been overridden since birth by other people's directions.

If the answer to 'why eat?' is boredom, depression, tension or loneliness, then find a more suitable solution than food.

How You Eat

The most common problem with the eating pattern is that overweight people eat too quickly. There is not enough time for the food to be digested and to reach the appetite control centre. So over-eating occurs. I remember having a meal and then being asked if I'd like some cheese. I really felt like it and so I answered yes. I was then called to the phone and when I returned I realised I couldn't possibly eat the cheese. In my 'pause' there was time for my appetite control centre to register that I'd had enough. Eating slowly is one of the most important things to do if you have a weight problem.

Eat from a small plate if you can as we do have a habit of finishing whatever is in front of us. If a large plate of food is given to us we will tend to eat it even while we protest that it is too much. If you have small children, feed them first, as getting up and down hinders the digestion.

Decide what amount of food is right for you, don't let others decide. I know this may be difficult but you wouldn't buy a pair of shoes and leave the shop without trying them on. So it is with the food requirement. If you eat everything that is given to you it is like taking the shoes which the shop assistant has chosen for you.

Focus on how you eat and what you are eating. Don't eat on the run. Sit down and make a meal of it. Don't eat while watching TV as your attention will be on the screen while you shovel food into your mouth in an unconscious fashion. Try and be as relaxed as you can at mealtimes; this allows the body to do its work properly without excessive emotions.

Learn to eat when your body needs it and stop when you have had enough.

What You Eat

Some foods will put more weight on you. You will know them from experience better than anyone else. Avoid or limit these. I know you will say, 'but I love them'. Unfortunately you have a choice – enjoy these foods or enjoy being slimmer.

There are many books by eminent dieticians advising on foods. I do not wish to enter this debate. There are obvious foods and drinks which contain so many calories it would be foolish to eat them except in minimal amounts.

Some people tell me, 'I'm fat because I just love food, I can't resist it.' I'm sure it's true that some people really do live to eat rather than eat to live. Just as someone who loves to drive at 100 mph has a greater risk of accidents than someone who drives at 40 mph. If they are prepared to take the risks and the complications then I don't feel they should hinder their desire, but they must accept that they will be overweight. It would be nice if we could have it both ways but, from my experience, 'Life ain't like that.'

Exercise

Obesity is the result of an imbalance between food eaten and the metabolism which converts the food to energy. It is like having a fire with too much coal – to reduce the amount of coal either put less on the fire or increase the flame.

There are many factors influencing metabolism and one is our attitude to our bodies. We have only one body and, as it has to last a long time, it is advisable to look after it. Just as we service a car to ensure it works efficiently so, to get the best from our body, we should devote some time each day to looking after it.

I believe it is important to spend at least 15 minutes a day doing exercise. Any form of exercise may be appropriate, but the type will vary with the person. It's not a lot to ask for your body. Swimming, jogging, exercising to music, skipping, brisk walking and cycling are all suitable. Include exercise in your daily routine – use the stairs not the lift, park the car some distance from the restaurant, get off the bus and walk some way to and from work. If it is possible to walk or cycle rather than using the car, do so. It is important to get into the habit of spending time on your body just as you spend time brushing your teeth to prevent decay.

The Mind

The mind plays a vital role in either maintaining obesity or ensuring weight loss. As I have stated, we often eat for our mind and use food to deal with emotional problems.

I believe that worrying about weight lowers the metabolism, hence less weight loss occurs. If you can stop weighing and stop worrying you are on the way to losing weight. People who get on and off the scales daily create a worry–eat pattern. I suggest you weigh yourself once every two weeks or not at all and just use your clothes as a guide to your weight.

Allow 20 minutes a day just for yourself and use self-hypnosis:

1. To relax and acquire a calmer attitude to the day's problems, which is an essential part in losing weight and keeping slim.

2. To understand previous emotions such as guilt, self-pity and anger, which may be involved in the weight problem – this is important in preventing the return of extra weight when future problems arise.

3. To build confidence and willpower, making a commitment to eat correctly and exercise each day – this provides an extra weapon in the 'battle of the bulge'.

4. To act as a substitute for food in lowering tension, giving comfort and enabling you to cope better with daily difficulties.

5.   To help you accept yourself, be yourself and like your-
     self, and therefore enabling your outdated attitudes
     involving food, such as, 'I'm no good, I'm fat and useless,
     I may as well continue eating', to be dispelled.

Positive attitudes are developed with the practice of self-
hypnosis and these, in turn, improve metabolism. I make
this statement not using scientific evidence, but from
observing many people who are able to deal with their
weight problem much more easily when they stop thinking
badly of themselves. Self-hypnosis is useful in decoding the
message the body is giving, both with the 'hunger' feelings
and with the message the excess weight is trying to give. It
may help you to understand how you became obese and how
the obesity is continually being maintained. It may also
be useful in diminishing the craving for sweet things pre-
menstrually.

Continuation of the eating directions we learnt when we
were young forms a habit-pattern which controls our intake
of food without the conscious mind questioning when,
where, how or why. This incorrect eating habit is what
causes all the pain and discussion about why 'we can't resist
food'. It may oppose how we 'ought' to eat and generally
wins the tug-of-war.

However, hypnosis has a role to play in reinforcing
willpower. Using statements such as, 'excess food is
poisonous to your body', 'your willpower will direct you away
from the fridge', 'you owe it to your body to look after it' or
any other phrase or statement which helps you alter the
pattern, will have more influence if repeated in a trance. This
is because the habit is being maintained by unconscious
forces.

Another way of helping to overcome the habit-pattern of

eating is to regard obesity as a disorder similar to diabetes. Diabetes is a disease of the metabolism in which the pancreas produces less insulin, and sugar is not metabolised properly. The diabetic patient, if not aware of this, becomes very sick and may die in a diabetic coma when the sugar level is very high. Diabetics need to regard themselves as different from others, and eat according to a special diet with limited carbohydrate intake. They may see others eating sweet things with no problem, feel annoyed, envious and may develop the 'it's not fair' attitude, but if they stray from the diet they will end up in hospital in a coma. So bitter experience dictates their behaviour and most learn to lead a full and enjoyable life within these limitations.

We could regard people with long-term obesity as having a similar metabolic disorder where, instead of a diabetic coma, obesity results if the eating pattern is not suitable for their specific metabolism. Obese people notice others eating sweet things with no problem but, unlike the diabetic, don't realise that they are different, and need to conform to their own eating pattern to prevent obesity. They too can branch out and eat what they would like but they are reminded of their inevitable downfall when a mirror is next passed.

Supervision

Another factor in maintaining weight loss is regular super-vision by a qualified person. Attending meetings gives an incentive to keep going with an eating programme. Aiming to lose a little regularly is much better then a 'crash diet', and support throughout this process can be very beneficial. In addition make sure you have an attitude of praise for the things you do rather than criticism for the inevitable mistakes. Being your own support is helpful when doubt and frustration raise their ugly heads.

To summarise what is an immense subject, I would suggest that to lose weight and maintain the loss a change in your present habits is necessary. Correction of faults in your eating pattern, your exercise programme and your mental attitude is important, as well as patience and persistence. The race you are running is a marathon, not a sprint, so keep in mind the necessary attitude required to complete it. At times you will fail and it is important to recognise this as a temporary failure, not an excuse to 'give up' and go back to the old, incorrect eating pattern.

My suggestion is to analyse some of your incorrect attitudes and habits, start a plan of action and tackle it on a day-to-day basis. Make a commitment for 24 hours only and, if some mistakes happen, don't give up just because you've gone off the rails; use these mistakes to reinforce your undertaking.

There may be people who are jolly and fat; I have not met too many. I have met many fat people who underneath are very unhappy and very keen to shed their excess weight and thus gain more self-confidence and self-esteem.

17

Phobias

Let me assert my firm belief that the only thing we need to fear is fear itself.

Franklin D. Roosevelt

I will show you fear in a handful of dust.

T. S. Eliot, *The Waste Land*

The definition of a phobia is 'an extreme, abnormal fear'. How does this exaggerated response to a situation come about? Sometimes the reasons are known, but most of the time there is no conscious awareness of the cause. Treatment may be directed to find out 'why', or to deal with the situation as it is in the present.

The fact that the phobic person is 'out of control' could be interpreted as being 'in the control' of the unconscious. There may be a protective or punishing aspect to this behaviour and hypnosis is often the treatment of choice to enable control to be restored to the conscious mind.

Almost any aspect of life may become fearful, as T. S. Eliot so aptly claims, and people who have one pronounced fear often have many others that are not so obvious. As hypnosis has a relaxing component it may be used in various ways to minimise the phobia.

In self-hypnosis, imagining the feared object or situation

at an immense distance, whilst feeling comfortable, provides a start to treatment. Being in control and allowing the situation or object to approach at such a rate that comfort can be maintained, help 'de-sensitise' the phobia. The time taken for this 'de-sensitisation' depends on the individual and it is important not to proceed too rapidly and cause panic. When, in a trance, the object or situation becomes close and the person feels at ease, it is time to proceed to a real-life situation.

Suppose you have a phobia of cats. This can be dealt with by imagining a cat at a distance and gradually bringing it closer in the mind with an associated calm feeling. When, in time, it is possible to picture the cat on your lap, then proceed to use a real cat at a distance.

Choose a friend who has a cat (preferably not vicious). Arrange for the cat to be in the next room with the doors closed. Achieve the relaxed feeling recalled from the trance state (see Chapter 5 for techniques). Gradually, with you in control of the cat's position and coupling notions of the cat with calm thoughts, arrange for it to be brought closer little by little. Having a peaceful scene in your mind helps to diminish the fear caused by the presence of the cat.

Phobias are irrational fears, for example:

Suzie was 40 years old and had an extreme fear of swimming. If her family went to the beach she would sit on the sand all day and swelter. All attempts to persuade her to go in the water failed and she had resigned herself to always being 'hot and bothered' at the beach, until someone suggested hypnosis.

I showed her how to relax and go into a trance and I asked her to practise this at home to gain some calmness when thinking about the sea.

When she returned she said she couldn't relax as the thought of the sea prevented her. I tried to help her imagine the water in the distance then her slowly walking down to it, but as soon as she got her feet wet she became very scared and opened her eyes.

We decided to explore the cause of her fear, and in a trance she recalled that when she was four years old she was swept out to sea by a strong current. She was terrified and swallowed a lot of water. Even though she was rescued in a few seconds by her father, it must have seemed like hours to her. I explained that this had happened a long time ago and that now she was older she could look after herself. I asked her to do self-hypnosis at home and to explain to the four-year-old 'in her mind' that she didn't need to be frightened of water.

Over a period of weeks she managed to control her unnatural fear and now goes for a dip in the sea, but she is still not too happy about taking her feet off the sand and always stays near the shore. Those few seconds of terror all those years ago have left an indelible mark on her mind.

Many people suffer from a fear of flying, which can be readily treated by hypnosis.

Tom is a 45-year-old businessman who has lost promotion due to his fear of flying. He has not flown since he was seven and always goes on holiday by car or boat even when it is very inconvenient. He also had another phobia which was fear of the underground train so I decided to see if we could deal with this first. We discussed whether these fears had arisen in childhood, but he had been through so many unhappy experiences that there did not seem to be one specific cause.

I taught him self-hypnosis and encouraged him to update his unconscious mind so that he was no longer reliant on childhood fears for safety. After a few sessions, when he felt comfortable, we went to his local tube station in London and spent some time going up and down the escalators. When he felt frightened we stayed at the top until he calmed down.

Next we sat on a stationary train and got off before the doors closed. We did this a few times, and then he put himself in a light trance and we travelled one stop. He got out, said he felt safe and so we travelled completely around the Circle Line with him becoming more confident with each stop.

Some weeks later we went through the process of imagining a flight – preparation, take off, landing, until he felt comfortable about making a journey. I told him to choose a short flight and let me know how it went.

A week later he rang me to ask if I would accompany him on a flight to Paris. I agreed and we met at Heathrow at 10 a.m. He was very nervous so we had a cup of coffee to discuss 'tactics'. I said we would buy the tickets on the condition that he could get a refund if we didn't fly.

At the booking desk I explained that I was a doctor and that Tom had a fear of flying. I asked the desk clerk if we could get a refund on our tickets if Tom was too frightened to board the plane. The man assured me we could get a refund and then I asked the time of the next flight to Paris. 'In 20 minutes, sir, but I wouldn't go on that plane – it's very narrow and if you have any trouble on the flight it's difficult to get out.'

That was just what Tom needed. He went as white as a sheet and rushed to the toilet. I thanked the gentleman for his help and waited for Tom to emerge.

Some cups of coffee later and after lots of discussion and cajoling, we boarded the plane and, apart from some white knuckles gripping the arm rest, all went well. We had lunch in Paris and Tom was in good spirits. Looking out of the window on the way back he said, 'There's nothing to it, why didn't I do this years ago?'

I, too, was very happy after a most satisfactory consultation, which resulted in my going home with some French bread and paté for dinner.

Frightening situations in childhood may leave an indelible mark in the back of the mind, suggesting the necessity for lifelong protection. As the child grows into an adult this protection is no longer necessary, but the fear remains with the same intensity as in the original incident. The child that is frightened holds on to the original terror as a warning to get away and this terror continues to recur in future non-threatening situations.

Jackie, aged 30, had had a fear of open spaces (agoraphobia) for ten years. The first incident happened when she found herself on a wide, open plateau while on holiday; she felt a terrible panic and rushed to a clump of bushes and hid in them until someone took her away in their car.

Since then the panic feeling had occurred on hundreds of occasions. She had tried many forms of help – tablets, acupuncture, psychotherapy, meditation – and received some benefit, but the condition recurred some time after treatment had stopped.

Jackie had grown up in a house full of tension. Her father was an alcoholic and was constantly frightening her mother or any of the four children who were within reach. All the family knew to keep away from Dad when he'd been drinking. Perhaps this held the secret of her fear of open spaces. Maybe to 'young Jackie' the need for a place to hide was life-saving, and her agoraphobia was really the child inside behaving as she did 25 years before.

As we talked about this possibility I noticed a glimmer of hope cross her face. I said that I would like to teach her self-hypnosis to get in touch with the 'young Jackie' and explain to her that things are often reversed in adulthood. Open spaces are much safer than hiding places, and her need to fear them was no longer a problem.

She cried a lot and talked about her fears that her father might hurt her, that he didn't love her, that she must have been a very bad girl for such terrible things to happen to her. With patience, time and understanding, the older Jackie reassured the young one. She said that there was no need to be frightened of father as he now lived in another country and couldn't hurt her.

After being in a trance for half an hour she opened her tear-stained eyes and said, 'I think she is going to need a lot of convincing,' then closed her eyes to rest after what must have been a most upsetting ordeal.

I explained that she should spend 20 minutes a day with 'young Jackie' talking, listening, understanding and letting her know it was going to be all right.

It took some weeks before the panic attacks began to subside. Many other problems in her life became evident and as she sorted them out the agoraphobia became less and less. She spent time communicating with 'young Jackie' and found it helped her confidence in many different ways; gradually, in her own time, she allowed the past to slip into the past where it belonged. She carried inside her a much happier and more peaceful little girl than she had previously.

If a situation can be interpreted positively or negatively, a frightened person will always choose the worst outcome as most likely. This is a form of self-protection and so it is very difficult to offer positive, logical alternatives for a phobic person who is in constant fear. That is why hypnosis, in dealing with the unconscious and avoiding the conscious, logical mind, is an easier, safer, more successful approach to the problem.

Claustrophobia and agoraphobia are very common. Many people are confined to areas around their houses that are 'safe' and panics occur when they feel 'out of control'. Going to the theatre or the cinema means booking a seat by the aisle; aeroplane flights are a nightmare; being a passenger in a car causes anxiety; motorways and even bridges are avoided if it all possible; invitations to gatherings and dinner parties where 'you can't get out' are refused and the thread of being in control dominates their life.

One researcher on the subject has again concluded that these instincts are remnants in our brain from our animal predecessors. An animal needs to be in control to avoid being killed by a predator. Open spaces (agoraphobia) provide a means to be hunted by the predator; enclosed spaces (claustrophobia) mean no escape from the predator. Hypnosis is a means of communicating with this ancient, deep part of our mind to update and reassure it that it is safe to be in these situations where control is not guaranteed.

Possibilities and Probabilities

During our daily life we automatically tend to divide events into two categories – possibilities and probabilities. Walking down the street we may be aware of the possibility of a brick falling on our head, but we don't dwell on that catastrophe as if it were a probability. We concern ourselves with happenings which have a likelihood of occurring and take steps to deal with those. If it is cloudy we may take an umbrella when we go to work. We allow time for a traffic jam on the way to the airport to meet a plane. These are all probabilities that require us to be concerned about their occurrence.

A person who has a phobia has somehow allowed possibilities to get into the probability compartment of the mind. Associated fears and worries are involved in a most unlikely event occurring. A fear of flying may involve excessive concern about the plane crashing. The rare possibility has become confused with a probability.

One way of helping such people is to guide their thoughts in a more appropriate direction. As the unnatural fears continue to dominate their minds they should say to themselves, 'Yes, it is a possibility that such and such will happen and I should worry proportionately but the probability is that it will not happen.'

These thoughts are directed to the unconscious mind during hypnosis, helping to bring logic into an illogical situation. Just reassuring the phobic person on a conscious level is unlikely to achieve the desired result.

Tony, a 45-year-old architect, had a fear of dying. He worried about this most of the day and tossed and turned at night fearful of dying in his sleep. Inevitably, his home life and work were greatly affected by his 'death phobia'. He had consulted many doctors and been prescribed sedatives, which helped slightly for a short time.

Four years previously he had been involved in a car accident and was nearly killed. This triggered off and

magnified the possibility of his dying and he had rumi-
nated on this thought ever since.

I talked to him about the fact that death was a
certainty, but when he would die was a matter of debate.
The probability was that he would *not* die today but there
was an extremely remote possibility that he might. He
should be less concerned about the one in a million
chance of a freak accident and more concerned about the
likelihood of living. I directed him to spend a suitable
amount of time being concerned about each of the two
eventualities. We also discussed the pity of wasting life in
worrying about death versus the likelihood that when
eventually he was about to die he would be concerned
with living.

Using hypnosis I directed similar logic to his unconscious mind and, applying post-hypnotic suggestion,
asked him to continue worrying a minute amount about
dying and use the rest of his energy for the problems of
living. When his fear occurred during the day he was to
recognise it as being acceptable but magnified.

Over the next few months he gradually apportioned
more of his time to living and became increasingly
involved in his work and home life. Strangely, when he
heard about death via the television or news, it seemed to
improve his attitude towards living. There were many
occasions when he dropped back into his old routine, but
fortunately lifted himself out by talking to himself about
possibilities and probabilities.

As phobias are about fears it is necessary to learn techniques
to relax as relaxation is the opposite of fear. Self-hypnosis is
a very good way to relax and using this technique on a daily
basis helps the mind to develop ways to feel comfortable.

This in itself gives control to the person who has a phobia.

Knowing you have the ability to relax is knowing you have a tool to overcome the enemy fear. It needs to be practised regularly so that when the need arises relaxation will be automatic. It is like a dress rehearsal before a play: the more you rehearse the easier it will be on the opening night.

The main aim with a phobia is to change your perspective so that a particular situation no longer triggers fear. The process of achieving this needs to happen in the unconscious mind – hence the benefit of hypnosis.

18

Smoking

Giving up smoking is easy. I've done it hundreds of times.
A patient

'You won't object if I smoke?'
'Certainly not – if you don't object if I'm sick.'
Sir Thomas Beecham, replying to a woman in a
non-smoking railway compartment

'To smoke or not to smoke?', that is the burning question. I wonder how much thought, money, energy, discussion and research are involved each year in smoking, its effects and how to promote or stop the habit. It's as if a battle is continually being waged between those who benefit from smoking and those who wish to eradicate the harm it causes. This battle is carried on in executive suites, laboratories and households.

In a social gathering if someone realises I use hypnosis in my medical practice two questions invariably follow: 'Does hypnosis work?', a question I find extraordinary having spent 20 years using it and promoting its benefits – I compare it to asking a chauffeur if he can really drive; and 'Can you make me stop smoking?', as if I have been waiting for this opportunity to test my skills.

I would like to discuss the use of hypnosis in helping people give up smoking under various headings, explaining methods, success rate and the likelihood of it being a suitable form of therapy. The discussion takes the form of a smoker's first consultation.

When Did It Start?

Smoking usually starts when teenagers try to be grown up. The cigarette is the symbol of adulthood. 'Keeping up with the mates' is a force which overcomes the taste, nausea and coughing spasms which accompany the first cigarettes.

Parents' smoking may set the standard for children to follow. The habit starts after a period of time and then no conscious thought is involved in the ritual of 'lighting up a fag'. An automatic response occurs after what was originally a deliberate act. Many so-called benefits are attributed to the nicotine, but most of these derive from the *belief* rather than the *chemical*. 'Cigarettes make me relax, feel more confident, give me something to do with my hands, help me to think better' are all comments in praise of the 'weed'. There are many reasons for initially giving a cigarette this false power:

- 'I started smoking when studying for exams 16 years ago and as I passed the exams I attributed my success to smoking.'

- 'I started smoking because I was nervous. The ritual of lighting up gave me something to do and I felt better. I am no longer nervous but the habit continues.'

So it goes on, starting as a matter of choice and then becoming habitual.

The Individual History

This gives an important assessment of the likelihood of success in stopping smoking.

1. 'Have you given up before and for how long?' If someone has given up previously for three months or more, this is a positive indication of the willpower required. If they have tried on numerous occasions and stopped for only a few days at a time, the motivation at this juncture will need to be very strong for success.

2. 'Does your partner smoke?' People whose partners continue to smoke may relapse quicker than those whose partners have given up or are non-smokers.

3. 'Why do you want to stop smoking?' If the reason is because someone else wants you to, the chances of success are minimal. Doing it for yourself is the necessary motivation. In my experience concern about health is more powerful than financial reasons.

4. 'Do you have children at home?'

5. 'How many cigarettes do you enjoy?' Most people enjoy five to six cigarettes during the day irrespective of how many they smoke. They have their 'favourite fags' – after coffee, first thing in the morning, after dinner, etc. If you smoke 30 a day and enjoy each one you are unlikely to give them up.

The First Challenge

When people ring to book an appointment to stop smoking, I ask them to cut down as much as they can for the 24 hours prior to the visit. This gives me an indication of their motivation and willpower. If someone stops completely for those 24 hours it's a very good sign. If they say, 'It didn't do any good, I smoked the same number as usual', it is obvious that they are not putting much of their energy towards stopping and are relying on hypnosis as the magic cure. I can assure you this is not the case.

It all depends on the smoker's attitude. They may say 'Let's get started, Doc. I've had my last cigarette and I'm ready to be a non-smoker.' or 'I'm still smoking and I really like it; I'm anxious about how I will be without a cigarette but I want you to stop my desire.' These are two different attitudes – one taking responsibility and requiring help, the other giving their problem to someone else to solve.

Hypnotisability

The majority of people (85 per cent) are capable of using hypnosis. Even people who are non-hypnotisable may benefit from the 'pep talk' the doctor gives – which can provide an altered attitude. Paying money to stop often helps, too.

Expectations

I discuss at length the intended way of giving up smoking with the person concerned. It is important to *stop*, not just to cut down. We work out an appropriate programme: some people prefer to reduce by a certain number a day or week; others feel better if they don't smoke after leaving my office. When the 'plan of action' is decided upon, I spend some time explaining hypnosis and correcting any false ideas or fears that are present.

I believe it is most important that each person is recognised as an individual, with a uniqueness about his strengths and weaknesses, his views and expectations. There are clinics where a pre-recorded tape is used and there is no personal interaction. A man came to see me after going to such a place. He had seen an advertisement for the clinic which claimed great success with stopping smoking. A receptionist requested £50, which he paid, and he was then shown into a room and told to lie down on a couch. The receptionist left the room and a tape recording about stopping smoking was played. He was so furious that as he left he 'lit up' to deal with his anger.

False Beliefs

There are many false assumptions made which the smoker continues to tell himself to legitimise his habit. These need to be discussed and corrected. 'Smoking relaxes me.' This may or may not be true. It is hard to imagine how nicotine, a stimulant, can relax, but the belief that it does will certainly create a relaxed feeling, so an alternative way of relaxing, using self-hypnosis, should be provided.

'Smoking helps me to feel confident.' If the smoker believes this then using confidence-building techniques during the self-hypnosis may replace the role of the cigarette. Sometimes smoking is a form of self-punishment for previous guilt. 'I'll smoke myself to death' is the unconscious message. Discussing this and bringing it to conscious recognition may enable it to be dealt with.

Danger Times and Forbidden Times

There are some times in the day when the smoking urge is very great. Each individual will know these times – on the phone, with a drink, at parties, after coffee, etc. These should be recognised so that 'forewarned is forearmed'.

There are some times or places where smoking is just not done. These show the capability of stopping and can be used to advantage. In church, in bed, in the bath, with mother-in-law, in a library, etc. The knowledge that you *can* stop for some time may be the basis of building the confidence to stop for longer and longer periods.

The Self-hypnotic Technique

There are a multitude of hypnotic techniques to help people stop smoking. There are aversive attitudes where the cigarette is directed to taste like camel dung (whatever that tastes like), and there are directive techniques where people are ordered to stop, with dire consequences if they do not. I am not in agreement with these approaches as I feel people should be encouraged to use a positive attitude in the direction of becoming a non-smoker.

Dr Herbert Spiegel, an American psychiatrist, is a leader in this field and has done much research to determine how effective his method is. He uses one session of 45 minutes, teaches his clients to use self-hypnosis and directs them to use his technique in a positive way.

He explains that the mind and body are two separate components and, as the mind controls the body, it is important for it to do so in a direction which leads towards health rather than away from it. A rapid induction technique which takes only a few seconds is taught and as the client drifts into a trance they repeat three sayings to themselves to diminish the urge to smoke:

1.   For my body smoking is a poison.
2.   I need my body to live.
3.   I owe my body this respect and protection.

In a very brief time 'the message' gets through and the client comes out of the trance. This can be done in public places without others knowing what is happening. Dr Spiegel explains that people wouldn't buy pet food if it had on the label, 'This food will poison your dog', and he suggests you should look after your body at least as well as your dog's. The point is to direct your thoughts in a positive way, 'Yes, I'll respect my body', rather than taking the negative approach, 'I won't smoke.'

   I will now relate an approach I use which involves relaxation and an altered attitude. I will recount a session with someone who had come to see me for the first time. The session was taped and the tape given to the patient to play twice daily at home. After a few days he was asked to see if he could achieve the same relaxation without the tape. He was to be seen once or twice again for reinforcement, depending on how he was progressing.

- Good. Allow yourself to get comfortable. Look up as high as you can, strain your eyes – that's right. Take a deep breath in. Hold it.
- Slowly let the air out and allow your eyes to close.
- Allow a drifting, floating feeling to develop in your body with each breath out. In your own time and in your own way, feel yourself floating down; time is

insignificant; don't try, just allow it to happen, all the way down.

[After about half a minute]

- Now use your imagination to walk ten steps into a garden, a lovely garden of your own creation, counting from one to ten for each step. Feel comfortable and secure there.
- Notice the trees, flowers, shrubs; notice the warmth, the sounds, the smells. Perhaps you can see and hear the birds. It is very calm and relaxing, peaceful and isolated.
- Feel the fresh air as you breathe it. Imagine how clean and fresh it is for your lungs and your body. Enjoy each breath and know you are using your body the way it should be used, the way it was made to be used.

[Half a minute silence]

- Now I want you to imagine how nature would be if all the things in the garden began smoking. Notice the smoky haze in the air, the brown nicotine discolouration of the flowers, petals and leaves, the smell of the flowers like a full ashtray.
- Look in the trees, notice the birds with cigarettes dangling from their beaks. Notice how they all sound like crows – no more beautiful bird-song, coughing instead. Notice the grass is brown and littered with cigarette butts.
- Notice how unnatural nature looks smoking. You are part of nature. You are as natural as the birds or the flowers. To your lungs you are acting as harmfully as the birds and the flowers would be if they smoked.
- Enjoy the garden as a *smoke-free zone*. Allow your lungs to be like the garden, to enjoy the natural air provided for them, without poisoning it with smoke.

- Spend the next few minutes enjoying becoming part of nature in that garden and make a commitment to keep it that way for the next 24 hours. Each day spend some time enjoying the smoke-free garden zone in your mind. Pay respect to your body which needs this protection to look after you for the rest of your life.
- When that commitment for the next 24 hours is agreed upon, then slowly leave the garden by counting from ten to one, keeping that good feeling of making a step in the right direction and come out of the trance in your own way and your own time.

The Enemy

There are many forces directing people to keep smoking. Friends offer cigarettes when they learn you are giving up 'the weed'. 'Go on! One won't hurt you!', as they wave the packet under your nose. It is a strange phenomenon and occurs also with obese people on diets and alcoholics trying to dry out. Perhaps it is jealousy; anyway, be forewarned.

Advertising on billboards, cars, sporting grounds and, magazines, promotes wonderful successes in all spheres of life and does its utmost to point out how masculine (or feminine) you are if you smoke a certain brand.

Success Rate

Assessing the success of any therapy for stopping smoking is very difficult. Unless a long-term follow-up is made, it is possible to have exaggerated statistics which are far from reality. People who stop after treatment may well go back to smoking three months later and the therapist will still count that as a success because he has no information to contradict this. Dr Spiegel's meticulous system for following-up his patients and his figures show an overall 40 per cent success rate over a period of years. This rate varies for different groups within this study, which demonstrates that the highest success rate is amongst people who are highly hypnotisable and are involved in loving relationships. Somehow this factor provided an increase in the willpower required to keep to the original commitment.

Giving up smoking is a very difficult task for some people; this is illustrated by a woman with arterial disease who was referred to me by her physician. He had told her that if she didn't stop smoking, the chance of her legs requiring amputation was very high. If she stopped, the arterial disease might not progress and she might save her legs. She continued to smoke 30 a day. I saw her on four occasions and no matter what I did or said she continued to smoke her legs away. I believe she was even smoking before they took her to the operating theatre. It's hard to understand but true; this woman preferred cigarettes to her legs.

So it is really up to you; it is your body and your decision. By having an attitude of respecting your body and realising that smoking is poisonous, you are taking a step in the right direction.

Remember: you can do it. When you were very young you were not a 'non-smoker', you were a 'free-breather', breathing the air that your body was made to utilise. You can achieve that attitude again, and using hypnosis will make the transition so much easier.

19

Dentistry

No passion so effectively robs the mind of all its powers of acting and reasoning as fear.

Edmund Burke

To most patients and many dentists, hypnosis is an enigma and a mystery. It owes its stormy history in part to the lack of a scientific explanation, even though no special skill is required to produce this altered state of awareness.

This chapter will discuss the use of hypnosis in dentistry and show how, once this art has been learnt, work on the teeth can become acceptable, even enjoyable. It has always been known that the teeth are the strongest and most durable part of the body. Given an unrefined diet, the biting surfaces wear slowly enough to last a lifetime and the forecast for the teeth of a Roman legionnaire or a sailor on the *Mary Rose* was invariably good.

This pattern changed completely when cane sugar was introduced into the diet. With a crystal refined to 99 per cent purity, a decay–abscess–loss sequence was started which became established for many generations. The desire for sweetness was satisfied at a terrible cost, not only in pain and suffering, but in early loss by extraction of the very component which should be the last to succumb to the ageing process. By contrast, compared with the natural teeth, a complete set of artificial dentures has an efficiency of something less than one per cent.

Today dentistry has reached a stage where the restoration of a decayed tooth is certain and long-lasting, where extractions are exceptional, where the skill of the dentist is matched by the excellence of his equipment and where the patient can expect to be treated with sympathy, kindness and understanding. However, a dentist waiting by his modern dental chair, new high-speed drill at the ready, local anaesthetic drawn up and a nurse waiting to be of assistance, are all of no use if the patient is cowering in the waiting room unable to move.

A normal fear of dentistry is very common and has some justification. Unnatural fear, where teeth rot and fall out due to lack of treatment, is a failure of great magnitude and an unnecessary loss of face (no pun intended) for the rest of the patient's life. Usually children are not frightened on their first visit to the dentist; the imprint of anxiety is stamped on the mind by an actual experience involving pain, blood or an intolerant dentist. It may have been the suffocating ordeal of an anaesthetic mask being forced over the small face of a screaming child. Such experiences remain in the back of the mind and act as a protective device to prevent a repeat performance. Unfortunately the knowledge of improved conditions, techniques and equipment does not reach this part of the mind.

If not a personal experience, then one related by a well-known and trusted person may create the fear. Such tales, exaggerated, harrowing and told in an over-enthusiastic way, can instil a terror of entering 'the bloody battle' with the dentist which can last for years. Any attempts at enlightening these frightened people with correct facts are seen as a ruse to lure them into a threatening situation. These stories may remain dormant and forgotten in the back of the mind until a dental problem triggers off the defence mechanism of fear. The fight or flight mechanism (see pp. 164–5) which occurs serves the purpose of keeping the person away from the dental surgery. It has been known for this reaction to happen when a patient is in the dental chair, and he will punch the dentist or run away.

The fear that people feel is shown in many ways, some more subtle than others – delay in making the appointment, changing the appointment time, arriving late, taking too long to remove an overcoat, frequent and prolonged rinsing and asking innumerable questions to delay the inevitable. Once the mouth is open and the dentist is 'in', further examples of anxiety are demonstrated by gagging, retching or vomiting, sweating, palpitations and overbreathing, perhaps even fainting.

This is where hypnosis plays a major role in converting a terrifying and unsuccessful dental appointment into a relaxed, acceptable situation. Compare the change in the following scenes and you will be able to appreciate the benefits of hypnosis, both to the patient and dentist.

Steve had a bad experience with a rough dentist when he was young and the resulting sense of terror has made him avoid dentists for 20 years. His teeth are in a foul condition, with many cavities and decay requiring urgent attention. Things get so bad – the pain, bad breath and difficulty in eating – that he forces himself to visit the local dentist, having a tot of whisky first, for Dutch courage. He sits in the waiting room, his heart pounding, his imagination running wild, hoping against hope that the dentist has been called away and that he will be sent home.

No such luck. His name is called and he marches stiffly into the dental surgery. He sits in the chair, grips the arm-rests tightly and hears, as if from a distance, 'Open please.' Feeling the sweat pouring down the back of his neck, he opens as widely as he can, but the tension is such that the dentist cannot examine his mouth properly.

'Relax, I'm not going to hurt you.' Steve hears only the word 'hurt' and tenses even more.

After some minutes of trying, the dentist puts his instruments down with a clatter and announces, 'I can't do anything. You're so tense it's as if you're the English goalie trying to stop a vital goal in the World Cup. You'll have to learn to relax.'

Steve breathes a sigh of relief as escape now seems possible. He listens to the lecture about the state of his mouth and the need to repair some of the damage. He is told he can learn to relax through hypnosis and, with or without the aid of relaxing drugs, have the dental work done with a minimum of discomfort. He realises that he can't continue as he is so he undertakes to learn to relax.

After a few weeks' practice he returns to the dental surgery, sits in the waiting room practising his self-hypnosis and waits to be called.

He is still nervous as he settles into the dental chair but is reassured nothing will happen until *he* is ready. Assisted by the dentist, he goes through the routine of relaxing and imagining a calm scene. He indicates he is ready by nodding his head, and local anaesthetic is gently injected and the dental work calmly performed.

You may feel this is a glib story which has been romanti-
cised to make it sound good. It is not so, and these scenes
which convert a nightmare into a daydream are repeated
daily. But there are many more scenes where the fear and
flight continue due to lack of knowledge of this form of
therapy.

A description of dental treatment with the patient in the
altered state of hypnosis might be:

> His eyes are closed, his breathing is slow, shallow and
> steady. His pulse is regular and firm. The muscles are
> relaxed, so much so that an arm lifted would feel heavy
> and limp and drop like a rag doll's. Suggestions are acted
> upon slowly, positively and without criticism. The patient
> appears to be 'miles away' and yet is willing to do as the
> dentist asks. The mouth and jaw muscles are relaxed
> allowing access to any tooth required.

The many qualities of self-hypnosis – relaxation, visual
imagery, dissociation, altered self-talk, analgesia – can be
used to help with dental phobia.

Julian, a 50-year-old barrister, had a problem with
gagging when he saw his dentist. It was explained to him
that the back of his throat was very sensitive and when the
dentist was working on his teeth the muscles in the back of
his throat contracted.

In order to help Julian with his problem I:

1. Taught him how to go into a trance and practise this
   nightly until he felt he had mastered the technique.

2. Showed him how to focus on a pleasant, relaxing scene

whilst in a trance and dissociate so that he felt he was there in his mind while his body remained in the chair.

3. Helped him realise he would be safe giving control to the dentist and that the muscles in the back of his throat did not need to be on guard to protect him.

Over a period of weeks Julian mastered these techniques, and with the co-operation of the dentist who allowed him to signal when he was ready, the dental work was completed in a most successful way.

Why then, if this is available to the population, are there so many people prepared to let their teeth rot rather than face the dentist? Is it the lack of education of the general public? Are there too few dentists practising and promoting hypnosis? Is there a general disbelief about the effectiveness of hypnosis or is the fear such that it won't even allow the thought of a dentist to be entertained?

Of the many attitudes prevalent in the community I will list a few which help to keep patient and dentist apart:

- 'I'm sure no one can hypnotise me.'
- 'I'm scared of what I may say when he gets me under.'
- 'I don't believe in mind over matter.'
- 'I'm scared of what he may find when he looks in my mouth.'
- 'I can't forget what happened when I went to the dentist when I was young.'
- 'How do I know it will work?'
- 'I'm too nervous to relax, I can never relax, it's not me.'

Other limiting factors are the number of dentists competent and interested enough to spend the extra time involved, and the lack of information available to people about dentists who do use hypnosis.

The specific uses of hypnosis in dentistry involve:

- Reducing the fear of pain and dentistry itself.
- Easing the discomfort of dental work by making the local anaesthetic more effective or even unnecessary.
- Allowing better relaxation for access to the mouth.
- Preventing gagging or retching.
- Minimizing bleeding following extractions.
- Lessening the fear of needles.
- Enabling the dentist to have first-class operating conditions.

Modern dental treatment has the advantage of a feather-like drill, quick acting local anaesthetics, sedative drugs if required and efficient filling materials. These are all used to the best advantage if the patient is relaxed.

If teeth and gums are not cared for they deteriorate and extractions may be necessary. The fear of dentistry is now generally unwarranted and the choice is between learning to relax or having false teeth.

To find out which dentists utilise hypnosis in their practice contact the Medical and Dental Hypnosis Society listed on p. 270.

20

Sleep

Sleep is the watering place of the soul to which it hastens at night to drink at the sources of life.

Abram Tertz

'Do you sleep well?' is a question asked in a medical interview. The answer tells a lot about the patient.

- 'Like a log; as soon as my head hits the pillow, I'm away.' This, as a rule, indicates the person is dealing well with the stresses of life.

- 'I toss and turn all night, my bed looks like a battle-ground', may mean inner turmoil relating to past or present events.

- 'I wake at 2 a.m. and can't get back to sleep', may be a sign of depression.

- 'I'm dead tired when I go to bed and I sleep for a couple of hours then wake up alert and can't get off to sleep', may indicate many unconscious factors playing a role in making certain he doesn't sleep.

To those who enjoy a good night's sleep its pleasure goes unnoticed; to those who struggle to obtain its benefits the long night is never-ending. Many curses, blessings, potions, pills and charms have all been directed to Hypnos the God of Sleep. Hypnosis was coined as a word when it was believed that an hypnotic trance was similar to sleep. It is not, but hypnosis has proved useful in treating insomnia.

Modern science has much research data about sleep patterns and problems. Sleep laboratories study people whilst they are asleep and monitor various physiological aspects of their mind and body. We now know a great deal more about the 'Brother of Death', and treatment varies considerably depending upon the problem encountered during the night. Generally insomnia is a symptom rather than the cause a problem. The mind is responding to some underlying factor either in the present or resulting from some past experience. Learning what these disturbing factors are will resolve the difficulty with sleeping. Often a habit is set up following some initial cause → response. The habit-pattern itself then becomes the cause for the insomnia.

Hypnosis is used to deal with either of these factors by: learning what is happening in the unconscious mind; and reprogramming it to overcome the habit-pattern.

Typical Features of Sleep Problems

I would like to discuss some important aspects of sleep problems in order to explain how hypnosis plays a role in their solution.

Some people sleep all night but wake tired and unrefreshed. This is because they do not reach a suitable depth of sleep, thereby not allowing the mind and body to benefit from the rest. This may be due to worry and anxiety from past or present events. The conscious mind does not 'let go' enough for the person to drift into a deeper state of sleep. Hypnosis can help to uncover past experiences causing anxiety, or to provide a way of 'turning off and relaxing' so that the tranquil state of self-hypnosis leads to a natural sleep of suitable depth.

We often fail to estimate the length of time we sleep. In hospital many patients claimed they 'hadn't slept a wink', but have been observed by the night nurse to have snored for many hours, not even waking whilst having their blood pressure taken. I was always amused to observe nurses waking patients to give them their sleeping tablets!

Trying to go to sleep is the best way of staying awake. Due to the need for a good night's rest, if we don't fall asleep within half an hour of going to bed, a pattern is set up which directs us to try to go to sleep. 'I must go to sleep or I'll be no good at the office tomorrow', directs the mind to be alert, and worry sends it in the opposite direction to sleep.

Hypnosis as a 'being' state rather than a 'trying' one can lead into a natural sleep. Using muscle relaxation followed by self-hypnosis, a tranquil, peaceful scene may be imagined and all thoughts of 'trying' fade into the distance.

A sleep tape made for the individual person can provide a suitable background to promote sleep. This is played in bed as the basis of self-hypnosis. Often patients complain they never hear the end of the tape as they have dozed off.

As children we may have said the prayer:

Now I lay me down to sleep,
I pray the Lord my soul to keep,
If I should die before I wake,
Pray the Lord my soul to take.

What a terrifying prayer for children to repeat before going to bed. The association between death and sleep is obvious, and has been remarked upon by poets since time immemorial. There is fear in some people's minds – either conscious or unconscious – that they may not wake up in the morning and hence by staying awake they stay alive.

Richard, a 25-year-old computer whizz-kid came to see me with insomnia. He lived on his own, was very intense, and was totally involved in his work. Two years previously he had been depressed, was seeing a psychiatrist and had spent time in hospital following an overdose.

He believed his insomnia became much worse after the overdose although his sleeping pattern had been very bad for five or six years.

In the first few sessions we talked about Richard as a person – his beliefs, attitudes, feelings, whether he still felt depressed, his relationships. He felt his attitude was much better now and his life was much more in balance. He was no longer depressed but still he couldn't sleep.

We discussed the conscious–unconscious connections and how they might be related to his symptom of insomnia. Richard agreed to use hypnosis and in a trance I questioned his unconscious about the cause of his insomnia. He relived the experience of the overdose, becoming very anxious and fearful as he described how black he felt, and recalling the words he said to himself when he woke in hospital.

'I could have died, I could have died.'

In that semi-stupose state he repeated this phrase again and again and in some way it became associated with sleep. The message his unconscious mind received was: 'Sleep could have killed me', instead of the more accurate message, 'Taking an overdose of sleeping tablets could have killed me.'

Our job was to disentangle 'sleep' from 'death' and it took many weeks for Richard's unconscious mind to be prepared to do that. He decided to practise self-hypnosis daily and when he went to bed changed the 'Sleep can kill' mantra to 'I need sleep to be alive and healthy.'

Changes did take place in the different levels of his mind and sleep returned – fitfully at first but eventually in a natural and healthy way.

Sometimes insomnia may be a form of punishment for some real or imagined guilt. Hence the saying 'the sleep of the innocent'. Using hypnosis to uncover the past experience and bring it to consciousness will allow it to be reassessed and a 'reprieve' obtained.

'Don't sleep on the job' may be taken literally by the unconscious mind. Someone striving to achieve in business or in other aspects of his life may, at some level, believe that staying awake will help him to be more successful. This, of course, is not logical and is not in the conscious awareness of the insomniac. He tosses and turns at night, ruminating about the activities of yesterday and tomorrow. He is very tired but as soon as his head touches the pillow he is alert.

The more he worries, 'I'll be tired tomorrow at work', the more sleep disappears over the horizon. The voice in the back of his mind saying, 'Sleep is an activity of the slothful', keeps him awake.

Using hypnosis to explain that sleep at night is not laziness and does not mean failure, helps to achieve inner peace which leads to a sound, restful sleep.

Past failures at going to sleep often awaken a self-fulfilling prophecy of 'I know I won't sleep again tonight.' Each night is a separate entity and lack of sleep one night has no relevance to the following night's pattern. Worrying about staying awake will most likely create that unenvied state. Using self-hypnosis as a routine at bedtime provides an avenue to direct the mind towards relaxation rather than involve it in worry and ruminations about previous failures. The very act of muscle relaxation and drifting into an altered state provides a restful bed where sleep can occur.

Sleeping tablets (hypnotics) are prescribed in their millions. In numerous cases they provide a suitable night's rest but often the sleep is not of the depth required, and the 'sleeper' wakes tired and groggy. They tend to have a habit-forming quality and may not produce a sleep pattern that is similar to natural sleep. Many people have great difficulty in trying to stop them.

If self-hypnosis can be learnt it removes any dependence on drugs, bolsters self-confidence and provides a natural sleep where the sleeper wakes rested and refreshed in the morning.

If you are tossing about in bed and not going to sleep it is important that *you get up after half an hour*. To stay tossing and turning means you are reinforcing your inability to sleep. When you get up do something – it doesn't really matter what it is – drink some hot milk, read a book, do some writing, watch TV, but stay out of bed for half an hour. In this way, you are breaking a cycle of not sleeping/worrying in bed. The bed should be for sleeping and if you are not, then get out of it, do something different and return.

Relaxation

The relaxing aspect of self-hypnosis (see Chapter 5) lessens any tension or worry which may be involved in the person's lifestyle or in his 'trying' to go to sleep. Many patients following a session of hypnosis in my surgery say, 'If I'd stayed in the trance a few more minutes I would have gone to sleep.' The trance state is so similar to the twilight state just before going to sleep that it directs the mind towards the tranquillity of sleep rather than to the alertness of the waking state.

Remaining in a trance state, even if sleep does not follow, provides the mind and body with many of their restful requirements. So if an hypnotic tape is played in bed and the person stays in a trance for some hours, he will 'wake' rested and refreshed.

A useful technique to induce sleep relies on the fact that 'trying to go to sleep is the best way of staying awake'. Conversely by distracting your mind to other subjects the process of sleep can take place unhindered.

It is preferable to have a routine you use every night that turns the process of going to sleep into a habit. Remember it is a natural phenomenon that occurs in every living thing, our aim being to help you get back in touch with this phenomenon rather than create a new method of going to sleep.

- Make sure you are comfortable, have been to the toilet and have finished your daily activities.

- Close your eyes and focus on your breathing. Do this for a few minutes noticing the regularity, the way it happens automatically, feeling you are the passive recipient of your breathing.

- Focus on the out-breath and associate it with a feeling of floating. Imagine a leaf floating down from a tree; imagine how that leaf feels.

- Notice different parts of your body relaxing as you focus on the floating feeling.

- Feel the change from an 'active attitude' useful in the day to a 'passive, not caring attitude' necessary for sleep.

- As you become more relaxed imagine a safe, comfortable, tranquil place where you would like to be.

- Imagine being in that place doing exactly what you want, knowing you are completely in charge and can alter it to suit your needs.

- Stay in that place maintaining a feeling of safety, comfort and relaxation and in your own time you will drift into a natural sleep.

We all have the ability to sleep. We have 'unlearned' that ability due to some experience or experiences in the past. Re-learning our ability to sleep may not require the sledgehammer tactics of nightly sleeping tablets with all their inherent defects. Perhaps learning to use your own resources to relax would be a more useful gateway to the Land of Nod.

21

Using Hypnosis to Build Confidence

The greatest thing in all the world is to know how to belong to oneself.

Michel de Montaigne

Hypnosis has been used in many areas of life to improve performance and self-esteem. Sports teams often employ a hypnotist to gain the maximum performance from their players. Exam candidates are taught self-hypnosis to retain facts and gain access to their memory. Businessmen learn hypnotic techniques to improve their sales results.

Self-confidence is a complex subject meaning either confidence in our ability to do things or confidence in ourselves as people. When we feel good about ourselves, we perform much better than when we are negative and self-critical.

Self-confidence comes about from a variety of factors including our genes, upbringing, parents, and experiences at school and during our teenage years. As we grow we develop belief systems which dictate how we feel about ourselves and others, how the world reacts to us, how willing we are to explore and take risks, and our activities at work and in relationships. Often these beliefs have no basis in reality at

all, 'I'm no good, no one likes me, I'll never succeed', may
well be an internal dialogue that is a complete fabrication.
This monologue may, however, create a self-fulfilling
prophesy that does indeed cause failure.

The underlying factors involved in confidence are:

1. What we say to ourselves – self-talk.
2. Memories of past events.
3. Internal pictures we form of either a past or future event.
4. Feelings – emotions related to specific situations.

Hypnosis is used to improve any or all of these components
and hence increase self-confidence. As we are often
unaware of the above factors it is necessary to use the trance
state to gain access to them and create a more positive
outlook.

Self-talk

- We tell ourselves negative things.
- We listen to ourselves and believe our statements to be facts.
- In following these apparent facts we feel bad.
- It is just as simple to tell ourselves positive things.
- When we believe and follow them, we feel better.

Listen to people commenting on themselves and you will
generally hear negative remarks.

- At a picnic, 'I'm so hopeless, I've forgotten the pepper.'
- At home, 'What's wrong with me, I can't even hammer a nail in properly?'

- At work, 'I must be going senile, I've forgotten to post that letter.'

Imagine making these comments about a child you know. How do you think he would feel if he was called hopeless, wrong, senile? He wouldn't feel great, proud or confident; he would not achieve his potential. So it is with self-talk; if it is negative it is limiting, detrimental and restrictive.

The aim of our internal dialogue is to support our needs, not destroy them. It should be tailored to the situations concerned and applicable, in a positive, supporting way, to you as a person. Having an attitude of 'Being your own best friend' is very constructive. Talk to yourself as if you are talking to your best friend, listen to your needs in a similar way. Use praise, optimism and care towards yourself and you will find that major improvements ensue.

Talking to yourself in a trance means that the messages have greater access to your unconscious. Affirmations (see Chapter 4) are a form of language used positively to 'brainwash' our minds.

As we grow up we develop different characters in our minds – the critic, judge, blamer – who cause fear, guilt and shame. We need to change those characters to become supporters, praisers and optimists so we can feel positive and hopeful about ourselves and our experiences.

When thinking about a future situation the phrase, 'Won't it be wonderful when...', points us in the right direction. When ruminating on past situations pick out the pleasant aspects and tell yourself, 'Wasn't it wonderful when ...' in order to produce contented feelings.

Improving self-talk can be useful in many situations (see Chapter 4).

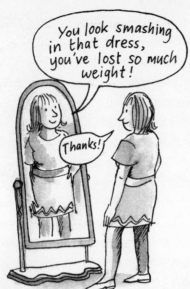

Having an attitude of being your own best friend is very constructive.

Memories

Our attitudes and actions are influenced by past experiences stored in the unconscious as memories. These memories become distorted with time and are not useful as a basis for attitudes and actions.

By reflecting on past experiences in a trance we can diminish the negative effect they have on our behaviour; we can put them into perspective for our present stage of life. They are stored with the intensity that they occurred originally and, as we have grown and developed many more strengths since then, they can be reduced to an appropriate level and the influence diminished.

David, a 40-year-old businessman, came to see me because he was frightened that as the best man at his friend's wedding he would have to give a speech. He had avoided public speaking all his life and the thought terrified him.

He remembered a time at school when he was ten and he had 'dried up' in front of the class whilst reciting poetry. He felt that was relevant to his present predicament. We talked about the various factors involved in his fear and he concluded that the following things were playing a role:

1. He was telling himself it would be a disaster, he would 'dry up' and everyone would laugh at him.
2. He had vivid memories of what happened at school and the feeling of not being able to speak properly.
3. He could see himself at the wedding making a complete fool of himself.
4. He had a sickening feeling in his stomach at the thought of the speech.
5. He had a desperate urge to avoid the whole wedding and pretend he was too sick to attend.

David and I discussed in detail his experience at school and his present situation 30 years on. We talked about the fact that all the people at the wedding were friends, who would support him. I also pointed out that most of the focus would be on the bride and groom. He agreed that the speech should be short and humorous and he had done a lot of homework to find amusing tales to tell about the bride and groom.

David then learnt self-hypnosis to help him relax, put the class experience when he was ten into perspective and implant positive messages to replace the negative ones.

He agreed to practise self-hypnosis daily and made his own tape recording in which he imagined the wedding scene, himself speaking freely and humorously and every-one laughing. He talked to the ten-year-old David and repeated the class-room scene until he saw it for what it really was – of no importance. He then created a warm feeling of liking himself to replace his fear and lack of self-esteem, by going over the positive things he had done in his life.

During the weeks before the wedding David became calmer and more optimistic about his role. His friends reassured him they were on his side and he realised he had blown the speech out of proportion.

The day went well, his speech was applauded, the few drinks he had beforehand helped and at our last session he said he might be able to do it again if necessary.

Creative Visualisation

People vary in their ability to form internal pictures – creative visualisation. Some see things almost as clearly with their eyes shut as open. Others form vague images, silhouettes, cartoon characters or nothing at all.

For those with vivid imaginations it is important that the pictures formed – either from the past or future – are relevant, helpful and appropriate. Often they are not and cause a lack of confidence due to the effect they have on thoughts and feelings.

Imagining ourselves as being confident and successful will help us to achieve that outcome. Creating a picture of gaining what we want causes a positive response from the numerous mechanisms running our thoughts and feelings. When looking for a parking spot if you imagine one in your mind you may be more likely to find one.

Reducing negative internal pictures, or increasing positive ones, will assist the variety of processes in the mind that create attitude and behaviour. Practising this in a trance has an even greater effect as critical judgement is diminished allowing the pictures to be more readily accepted. As the saying goes, 'One picture is worth a thousand words.'

Feelings – Emotions

Emotions are the most powerful influences on our behaviour. They override thoughts in the majority of situations. 'We are what we feel' may be a good description of us as human beings.

Patients come for therapy because of their feelings, 'I feel sad, frightened, depressed, angry, guilty, etc.'. Very few patients come with the complaint 'I think ...'.

As feelings are the main problem and the most powerful force, it is important they are on your side, working for you and with you, up to date and suitable for your specific needs. All too often we carry feelings from the past and project them into the future. They are stored as memories and triggered by thoughts or experiences. They may try to be protective but in fact are restrictive or destructive.

One thing I would like to say with great conviction is that feelings are not easy to change. They have a life and mind of their own. We can alter thoughts by using a process of rationalisation, but saying, 'Don't worry', to yourself, for instance, either has no effect or creates the reverse of what is intended.

Feelings require subtle influences and frequently the passage of time to help them change. The trance state is very useful to gain access to feelings stored in the body and we can then develop a healthier perspective on these feelings in relation to our present situation.

A technique where the 'adult you' talks to the feeling which is representing the 'child you' helps to release out-of-date emotions and replace them with adult ones (see Chapter 10).

Jennifer had led a troubled life ever since she left her parents five years before she consulted me. She was 25 at the time of her visit and wasn't coping well with the world and its challenges. 'I've always been shy and terrified of taking risks', was the way she described herself.

Early experiences of failure and criticism had forged an imprint in her thoughts and feelings, so she created a motto for herself, 'Avoidance is safest', and followed that rule in any interaction she had. Whenever there was a choice in her life, Jennifer chose to opt-out and say 'No'. The fact that she was alive and healthy reinforced her attitude as being the best possible.

She came to see me because she realised life was passing her by. Everyone seemed to be having a better time than she did. She wanted to change but didn't know how.

We discussed confidence and what it meant to her; the internal factors playing a role in her perspective on life; hypnosis and how it might be of help; and the time it might take for her to change. She agreed to see me every two weeks for six months and we formulated the specific outcomes she wanted to achieve.

Jennifer worked very hard at the tasks I set and practised self-hypnosis daily. My main focus was to encourage her to take risks and not worry so much about the outcomes. I told her it didn't really matter if she was successful or not as long as she learnt something from the experience. I pointed out that avoidance teaches very little.

Throughout the six months her feelings changed little but she followed the edict 'feel the fear and do it anyway' and was pleasantly surprised she was able to do so. She was still having difficulties but felt she had learnt a great deal about the components that were causing lack of self-esteem and how to install new ones that would help her confidence grow. She learnt to talk to the 'little Jennifer' inside and be her friend and guide. She was able to focus on positive aspects of herself, life and future outcomes.

The role of hypnosis and self-hypnosis in confidence is that it enables us to implant ideas, pictures, words and perspectives into the deeper levels of the mind where the foundation stones of confidence reside, thereby creating a more positive attitude, towards both ourselves and the situations that confront us daily.

22

Hypnosis and Children

A child is a flame to be kindled not a vessel to be filled.

François Rabelais

One of the aspects of hypnosis that is so useful as a therapeutic tool is the ability to suspend critical judgement in a trance. If I say to someone in the conscious state, 'You are on a beach', the reply could well be, 'Don't be daft, I'm here with you in this room; have you gone mad?' In a trance the response may be, 'Yes, it is lovely and warm and I can hear the sound of the waves as I lie on the sand and I also know I am here with you.'

The trance state has enabled the person to accept suggestions without the analytical part of the mind being involved. Children have this facility naturally; their imagination plays a major role in their lives. If you say to a child, 'Close your eyes and see two dogs playing', they will describe the dogs and their activities in detail.

Using hypnosis with children is very easy and very rewarding. Because they accept suggestions less critically than adults they respond well to this technique. As children

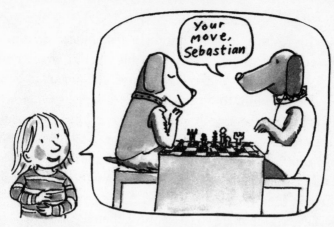

If you say to a child "Close your eyes and see two dogs playing" they will describe the dogs in detail and the activities occurring between them.

grow up they lose much of this 'uncritical acceptance' and hypnosis needs to become more subtle to avoid conscious interference. Many childhood conditions respond well to hypnosis – bed-wetting, nail-biting, asthma, eczema, fears and phobias, bowel problems, nightmares and sleep disturbances, tantrums and emotional outbursts.

Because the child's inner world is so vivid it responds to creative visualisation (see pp. 65 and 243). I have used this method with children for many years and am always pleasantly surprised at the way they respond and the rapidity with which they form pictures. This inner world does not have any logic and is full of symbols and metaphors of the child's creation. Using this technique means that the therapist is on the child's wavelength and communication is greatly improved.

If a child complains of a 'pain in the tummy' we may use adult words to describe it as abdominal pain, constipation, etc. If we move into the child's world and ask him what he sees in there he may describe 'a yellow string tangled up'. This is his real inside world and if, instead of leading him to adult terminology, we continue on his level he may say he wishes to 'untangle the yellow string and make it blue'. When we help him to do this his pain disappears.

Visualisation is a technique I have encouraged many mothers to use with their children – from the age of five to young adults in their twenties – with remarkable success. The aim is to use the child's imagination and to change the pictures in their internal world.

Because children are so susceptible there is no need to go through an induction process. It is important to gain their trust and generally I have a parent sitting in the room for reassurance. Asking a child to 'close his eyes and go inside' is enough to have him engage in his internal world in such a way that suggestions for change are readily accepted.

The child certainly does have an ability to resist ideas that are not acceptable and will come out of his world in order to maintain control. It is very important to use 'clean language' where the adult is not imposing his or her beliefs on the child. This form of language directs the child to explore attitudes and thoughts so he is free to utilise his own creative world to make changes. Using words like 'should', 'must' or 'ought to' will cause him to realise he is in adult territory and his flow of internal activity will be restricted. Encouraging him to work in his own way, and supporting him in the process, will allow him to make suitable changes to the internal pictures.

Suzanne, a bright ginger-headed ten-year-old, was frightened to go into her science class. Neither she nor her mother were quite sure how this had come about but she had complained of a sick feeling and had to leave.

During the previous term she had been able to do science, on only two occasions. She was fine with all her other classes but was falling behind in science, causing concern for both parents and teachers.

I asked her to 'go into' the sick feeling and tell me what she saw.

'It is hot and round and yellow and it doesn't feel nice. It is in my tummy.'

'And when you go to the other classes and feel well, what is it like in your tummy then?'

'It is much cooler and green and it doesn't have a real shape.'

'Are there any sounds or voices in your tummy with the round, hot, yellow feeling?'

'Yes, I am telling myself I must go into the class or I'll be in trouble and fail my exam.'

'And when the cool, green shape is there, are you saying the same thing?'

'No, it is quiet then.'

I asked her to practise going in and out of the science class to learn about the change from green to yellow. Even if she stayed only a few seconds, that would be fine in order to discover what triggered the change.

The next time I saw her she said she believed the smell of gas in the class may have caused the change of colour. She remembered a time at home when there was leaking gas and the man who came to fix it said it was very dangerous. Her mother confirmed that there had been a leak and perhaps Suzanne had picked up the sense of danger in the household.

Suzanne and I talked about the incident and the smell from the Bunsen burners at school. I helped her realise that this smell was not dangerous. We continued talking until I felt Suzanne was able to recognize the difference between the two situations.

Suzanne was soon able to have the quiet, green feeling when she went into the science room even if there happened to be a smell of gas present. She continued to focus on that feeling and was able to resume her science lessons again.

Most feelings can be visualised by children.

Rosie was a sensitive 12-year-old who was very frightened of staying at anyone's house overnight. All her friends went to 'sleep-overs' and the fact Rosie was unable to join in was becoming a major focus of attention for her family.

I talked to both Rosie and her mother. I then asked Rosie to imagine her fear and to tell me how she felt when she was invited to stay at a friend's and where the unpleasant feeling was situated. She said it was in her tummy so I asked her to close her eyes and go inside her tummy and tell me what the feeling looked like.

'It's like butterflies flying around.'

'Are they large or small?'

'They are pretty and coloured and moving very fast.'

'If you were feeling happy what would that feeling be like?'

'It would be calm and blue and in my tummy.'

I asked Rosie to think of a happy time and let me know when she had the calm, blue feeling inside. I asked her to try and keep the calm feeling and imagine she was going to stay at a friend's house. But she said the image moved to the butterflies again.

I asked Rosie to open her eyes and then we discussed

what I wanted her to practise at home over the next week. Each night Rosie was to spend a few minutes imagining going to a friend's and changing the butterflies into the calm, blue feeling. It wasn't easy, but eventually Rosie was able to do this. She then decided to try out the technique for real and she stayed over at a friend's for the first time in her life.

When she came to see me Rosie proudly described how she had gone to her friend's house. Every time the butterflies started to come she had concentrated on the calm, blue feeling until she fell asleep.

Children have an advantage over adults in that their ability to use imagination is unhindered by logic or reality.

Creative visualisation is an amazingly easy, powerful and quick way of using internal imagery to help children overcome problems. The source of its power is that it involves the child's perspective and feelings being represented as pictures. In this way logic, analysis and adult attitudes are avoided and progress – often rapid – is made as pictures change causing a great improvement in feelings.

23

Post-traumatic Stress Disorder

The most powerful emotion of all is fear; it robs us of any positive attitude or intention.

Brian Roet

Post-traumatic stress disorder is a verbal mouthful describing a very simple concept – after an upsetting incident we feel terrible. When this unbearable feeling lasts longer than expected, treatment is required in the form of therapy; hypnosis is very useful as part of this treatment.

The individual components of post-traumatic stress disorder are:

1. An extremely traumatic, even life-threatening, event occurs or is witnessed, causing panic, and a feeling of helplessness and loss of control.

2. The person continually re-experiences the event and avoids anything associated with what happened.

3. A state of anxiety is maintained plus an attitude of alertness which reduces the ability to enjoy things as before.

4. There is a loss of interest in life and a numbness or detachment from others as if they don't understand.

5. These symptoms last more than a month and require help to be resolved.

The mind acts differently when involved in situations threatening our survival. It sets up a mechanism aimed at protecting us from a similar event in the future, but often causes problems rather than giving solutions. Emotions involved in post-traumatic stress disorder may be fear, anger, guilt, frustration, depression or anxiety – all related to the initial incident. This incident may have occurred in adulthood and be remembered, or in childhood beyond conscious recall; in this latter situation the patient experiences the intense emotion but is completely unaware of its origins.

A sequence of events may be:

1. A robber appears at a teller's window wearing a balaclava and brandishing a gun. He demands money.

2. The teller is terrified believing he may be killed. He hands over the money and the robber runs out of the bank.

3. Pandemonium ensues; the manager and police are involved. The teller is questioned and allowed home.

4. At home he explains what happened and starts to shake. He has a fitful night disturbed by nightmares.

5. The next day he is unable to return to work, feels terrified and starts to experience panic attacks.

6. Over the following weeks he attempts to return to work but feels panicky and is unable to do so believing his life is in danger if he starts work again.

This situation continues until he is referred for therapy. It is important that counselling begins as a debriefing within two to three days of an incident to stop the build up of fear and anxiety. In this way the internal workings of the mind can be assessed and help provided to prevent a long-term problem.

Looking at the above components: when the robber appears at the window, the teller would experience an intense feeling of panic. The words 'I'm going to die' are the most drastic any living organism could hear; they cause all the systems in the body to go on to 'survival alert' – hormones and adrenaline are released, the heart races, muscles tense, the nervous system sends thousands of messages around the body, the brain becomes intensely focused, and an imprint of the robber and what he said is formed in the mind.

This intensely stressful incident alters the equilibrium of the teller preventing his emotions from settling down and returning to their previous state. At some level he remains on high alert for future danger. The sight and sound of someone similar to the robber may trigger off a panic reaction, as may returning to the scene of the crime.

How can a therapist help the teller return to normality, and how is hypnosis involved? The technique used to help post-traumatic stress disorder involves:

1. Giving quality time to the patient, allowing him to talk about the incident and his feelings. Attentive, supportive listening is a very powerful tool in these situations.

2. Affording him time away from the original situation so his emotions can settle down.

3. Teaching him relaxation techniques to restore order to his nervous system.

4. Helping him to go through exactly what happened slowly (facts, thoughts, feelings), focusing on every detail until he was safe after the incident. This needs to be repeated over time until he can describe the sequence of events without fear. In a trance it is possible to do this and regulate emotions during the process. It is important to be sensitive and avoid worsening the experience. (Some people call this the 'horror movie technique', based on the fact that if you repeatedly go back to view a horror movie, eventually it will become boring, the fear being removed by repetition.)

5. When he feels ready, helping him to go back to the scene of the crime in such a way that he can leave if fear recurs.

6. Allowing time for the healing process to take place.

7. Using hypnotic techniques to resolve any fear stored in the unconscious.

It is said that our memory plays tricks on us and in part that is true. My model is that the memory functions in three separate ways:

• **Category A:** We forget experiences. I call this 'allowing time to go into the "forgetory"' (a name I have given to the place where things go when we forget them). If we try and recall what we had for lunch three months ago we will be unable to do so – that fact is in the 'forgetory' as it was not considered important enough to retain.

• **Category B:** We can remember incidents as facts. If we fell off a bike and hurt ourselves when we were very young, we may be able to recall the incident but associated emotions have been removed with time. This is called 'factual memory' as it involves only the facts of the experience.

- **Category C**: If an incident is remembered in an emotional way it is called an 'emotional memory'. Recalling the event produces emotions similar to those that occurred originally. Time passing does not diminish their intensity as with less traumatic experiences.

The aim of therapy is to help detach emotions from the memories of traumatic incidents. Techniques used remove memories from Category C and replace them in Category B.

Noel is a 36-year-old housewife, happily married with a six-year-old son. She was referred to me because of her fear of shopping in the supermarket. Three years previously she had been waiting in the check-out queue when a drunken woman had accosted her. During the scuffle she fell, breaking her glasses and causing her nose to bleed.

Since that time she had been unable to go into the supermarket and her husband had taken over. Three months ago he changed jobs and his hours of work made it difficult for him to shop, so Noel decided it was time to do something about her fears.

We spent the first two sessions discussing her problem in detail. I explained to her the concept of post-traumatic stress disorder and the three forms of memory involved. I suggested we needed to change the memory of the incident from Category C to Category B and we would use hypnosis to help. I taught her self-hypnosis and asked her to practise daily at home. When she returned she demonstrated her ability to go into a trance.

While she was in a trance I asked her to imagine three containers in her mind: A – on the left – the 'forgetory'; B – in the middle – the 'factual memory'; and C – on the right – the 'emotional memory'.

She nodded as she saw the pictures in her mind, and said 'I can see them – the left one is black, the middle one is blue and the one on the right is yellow'.

I continued, 'There is someone in your mind who decides in which container to put your past experiences. Can you imagine seeing that person?'

After a little while she nodded and told me he looked like a judge with a gown and wig. We then established that he was responsible for putting memories into the different containers. I told Noel to let him know that the memory from the supermarket was still stored in the emotional memory container and was causing problems, and to ask him to put it in the middle factual container. A little while later she nodded to let me know he'd done this.

I asked her to recall the incident and describe it to me now. 'It's much better. I can see what happened but it is as if it happened to someone else.'

'Now I'd like you to see yourself in the future, going into the supermarket shopping calmly and comfortably.'

She sat quietly for some time, her face placid and relaxed.

'Yes, I can do that and I feel OK.'

When she came out of the trance, she was very enthusiastic. She agreed to continue to practise self-hypnosis daily, making sure the memory stayed in the factual container and imagining herself successfully going shopping.

When I saw her two weeks later she had made a number of attempts to shop in the supermarket. At first she had to leave but eventually, after two months, she was able to shop as she had before the incident.

Traumatic experiences do not have to be as drastic as the above to cause problems. When we are children – vulnerable and powerless – things happen to us which on the surface would not seem traumatic at all. Due to our sensitivity, words, actions and attitudes take on special significance and may cause stress for a long time afterwards.

Fears, however irrational, originate somewhere at some time due to some situation. We may not be able to remember the incidents but the emotion is there linked to the 'unknown' experience.

I saw a man who was terrified of snails. Every time he thought a snail might appear on TV he turned off the set. He couldn't watch or listen to gardening programmes and he had no garden of his own.

He had absolutely no idea how he had learnt to be terrified of snails. He stated he had been frightened for as long as he could remember. His parents were dead so we couldn't explore that avenue.

Under hypnosis he reported coming home from school as a four-year-old and a group of older boys putting a handful of snails down his neck. He had completely forgotten, or repressed, this memory and only recalled it using recovering techniques in hypnosis.

Once he had brought this traumatic memory to his conscious mind he was able to reduce its influence. He moved it from the 'emotional' to the 'factual' container, and by utilising self-hypnosis daily for two weeks was able to hold a snail in his hand without fear.

Using a variety of techniques in hypnosis we can regress patients to forgotten experiences. In this way we can learn about the original situation and assess if it is still helpful to carry those emotions into the future.

The concept is that 'we know but don't know we know'. Uncovering techniques help this knowledge to move into our conscious awareness. Sometimes patients are surprised at what is uncovered; at other times they say they were vaguely aware of it anyway.

Sandra had an aversion to chocolate. At the age of 35 and with two children she made up her mind to tackle her problem and came to see me for help. She complained that it was difficult to get through the day without some contact with chocolate.

Sandra's history involved being sexually abused by her father from the age of 10 to 14. She had received long-term therapy and was coping well with her life in every respect. She was not sure if the chocolate phobia was related to her abuse and believed hypnosis would help solve the problem.

After three consultations we decided to use a technique called the 'Affect Bridge' where a feeling is traced back in time and the patient remembers a similar sensation at younger ages until the first time it was experienced. We literally use feelings to bridge the preceding years.

Sandra's feeling was an intense nausea in the middle of her stomach at the sight or smell of chocolate. I asked her to close her eyes and focus on it. She sat quietly and indicated that she was in touch with the feeling. I then told her I would count backwards from 35 through the years. Each time she felt that feeling and recalled an associated incident she was to raise a finger. As we came close to 14 her finger suddenly moved and she started to cry. Her body shook and she opened her eyes.

'It was him. It was him all along. I saw him. I saw him giving me chocolates after he did it.' She convulsed in tears and was unable to talk.

After a few minutes, staring into space and talking in an automated way she went on, 'How could he do it? How could he do it to a little girl and just walk away?'

Sandra had uncovered the connection. Her father had given her chocolates after abusing her. This fact had been lost to her memory but the emotional connection still remained. The chocolates symbolically represented the violation and the sight or smell of them triggered off the intense feelings of nausea.

Sandra and I spent many sessions dealing with the events that she reported. With great difficulty she learnt to place them in the factual memory container. Her aversion didn't disappear completely as the experiences had been too traumatic and too repetitive. She accepted what remained of her chocolate phobia and was at peace now she had discovered its origins.

Trauma therapy is a vast subject and can be applied to many of the problems seen by psychotherapists. The healing process requires time and support as well as the many hypnotherapeutic techniques used to restore peace and tranquillity to the troubled mind.

24

Questions About Hypnosis

If we can really understand the problem the answer will come out of it, because the answer is not separate from the problem.

Krishnamurti

Over the years I have been asked many questions about hypnosis, self-hypnosis and hypnotherapy. The following are some of the most common.

Q: *Can anyone be hypnotised?*

A: In the clinical setting most people who want to be hypnotised can be hypnotised. As hypnosis is a co-operation between therapist and patient it is necessary for the patient to trust the therapist before allowing himself to go into a trance. Some people go into a deeper trance than others depending on what is called their 'trance capacity'. This is made up of many factors – genetic make-up, state of mind at the time, ability to let go, need to be in control.

Q: *If I can be hypnotised easily does that mean I am gullible and of low intellect?*

A: No. Hypnotisability and intellect are unrelated. It is true that those with a very low IQ may have difficulty in being hypnotised if they are unable to remain focused for long enough to go into a trance. The more feeling, creative, imaginative and artistic you are the more likely you are to 'let go' and enter a trance. The more thinking, controlled and frightened you are the less likely.

If you are a thinker, you may tend to analyse what the therapist is saying; if you are emotional, words will be transposed into feelings and you can let go and drift into a trance.

Q: *Could I remain in a trance and not come out of it?*
A: No. The trance state is a natural one and if you were left in a trance by the therapist, you would either come out of it or go to sleep and wake naturally.

Q: *Will I say or do something I don't want to when I'm hypnotised?*
A: No. It is in the interests of therapy to utilise the trance state to help the patient. If the therapist asks questions that are upsetting the patient, he will either come out of the trance or refuse to answer. A sensitive therapist should notice the patient's body language, be aware that a conflict is arising and avoid similar questions.

Q: *Is hypnosis available on the National Health Service?*
A: Many practices are starting to employ complementary therapists to assist medical treatment and some employ hypnotherapists but at present these practices are in the minority.

Q: *How would I know if I was hypnotised?*

A: There are many signs of being in a trance but none is infallible. The popular concept that you go to sleep, are unaware of what is happening, and wake up cured, is quite incorrect. Most people say they are relaxed, can hear everything but feel so comfortable they are happy to stay sitting with their eyes closed.

They will have a focused attention on what the therapist is saying, perhaps have parallel awareness – being in the consulting room and somewhere else as well – and experience time distortion – a half hour trance feels like ten minutes. There will be a dream-like quality to the session. They may recall events from the past, and hopefully see things from a different perspective.

Q: *Is hypnosis useful in the treatment of asthma?*

A: Yes. Many medical references describe the benefit of hypnosis for asthma – especially in children. Stress is often involved in asthmatic attacks so that relaxation is of significance; visualisation helps the patient to see wide bronchial tubes with air easily flowing in and out; reducing the fear of an attack may help to reduce the attack itself. Self-hypnosis, relaxation and visualisation techniques all help asthmatics. Hypnotic training should be used in conjunction with medical supervision of the asthma.

Q: *Is hypnosis useful for bowel problems?*

A: Yes. Research has shown that the bowel is a much more sensitive organ than previously thought. There are many more nerve endings and connections with the brain than we realise. Because of this, the mind–bowel connection creates major responses from emotional causes.

Recently medical journals have published scientific papers showing the benefit of hypnosis in irritable bowel syndrome. This condition shows no organic pathology on X-ray but causes symptoms of pain, bloating and swinging from constipation to diarrhoea. Using hypnosis these symptoms are often cured.

Q: *Is being hypnotised the same as being asleep?*

A: No. The trance and sleep states are very different. When you are asleep you are unaware of what is happening around you; in a trance you can hear what the therapist says, and also extraneous noises, but are able to remain relaxed rather than be disturbed by them.

If you listen to an hypnotic tape and come out of the trance when the therapist tells you, this means you were definitely in a trance; if you remain still for an hour after the tape finishes you were most likely asleep.

Q: *Will I be under the control of the hypnotherapist?*

A: No. This is impossible. As previously stated the aim of therapy is for the therapist and patient to work together towards a positive outcome. Co-operation is achieved by the therapist offering useful suggestions in the trance, the patient feeling safe and secure enough to accept them. If the patient feels he is losing control he will increase his resistance and the benefits of therapy are reduced. By relaxing and letting go he will open his mind to the therapeutic comments of the therapist. If at any time the patient feels threatened or unsafe he can come out of the trance and express his concern.

Q: *Does it take a long time for a therapist to hypnotise someone?*

A: No. The induction of hypnosis varies from therapist to therapist. Some have a routine lasting 20 minutes, others only five. The basic components are focused attention, eye closure, and the therapist's monotonous voice guiding the patient into a deeply relaxed state.

    As it is a natural phenomenon, it is really only necessary for the patient to trust the therapist and allow it to happen, and for the therapist to avoid suggestions or tones of voice that will prevent the patient going into a trance.

Q: *Can hypnosis help us to remember experiences previously forgotten?*

A: The answer is yes and no. Hypnosis can certainly aid recall and bring to consciousness events that were forgotten. Patients can also 'remember' things that didn't actually happen. It is just as easy to make up something in a trance as it is in the conscious state. Some years ago hypnosis was used in the police force to solve crimes; now it is recognised that the benefit from hypnosis is minimal. The facts remembered in trance were frequently found to be incorrect. The witnesses were unintentionally making things up to please the hypnotist or the police force.

Q: *Do you always have success when you use hypnosis?*

A: No. Like any form of therapy there are many factors involved in whether the patient achieves his aims or not. As I have previously mentioned the most important elements are motivation and time and effort on the part of the patient. Many symptoms are not suitable for hypnotherapy just as many illnesses require specific tablets.

Q: *If I have been hypnotised in therapy will I change my personality and become a different person?*

A: No. Being hypnotised will not alter your personality. You may gain an insight that allows you to choose different alternatives, but you as a person are not changed. Sometimes, however, relationships change, for instance, when the patient realises he has been treated like a victim by his partner. If he chooses to become more assertive it may disrupt a previously dysfunctional relationship. This doesn't mean that hypnosis has made him a different person, it means he has learnt to see the relationship from a different perspective and has chosen to alter it.

Q: *If a stage-hypnotist can make someone eat an onion and think it is an apple, could hypnosis cure people just as quickly?*

A: No. Actions on stage cannot be duplicated in therapy. I spoke at length to a stage-hypnotist on this subject and he reminded me that the settings are very different and the responses not comparable. Stage-hypnosis encourages extroverts; therapy generally attracts more introverted people. Stage-hypnosis is aimed at entertainment; clinical therapy aims to solve problems and change attitudes. Stage-hypnosis is for a short, two-hour span; therapy is for long-term change.

Q: *How long does hypnotherapy take?*

A: As each person is different it is hard to assess how many sessions are required. Hypnotherapy aims to be brief compared with analysis. It is a good idea to negotiate a set number of consultations with the therapist and re-negotiate when these have taken place.

A number of factors are involved in deciding how many sessions are needed – personality of the patient, history, present situation, symptoms, hypnotisability, attitude, etc. It is useful to be aware of the progress of therapy and discuss the situation if it is not heading the way you intended.

Many questions arise when hypnotherapy is contemplated. It is important to recognise whether or not these questions are preventing you from seeking help and to have them answered satisfactorily so you have peace of mind if you decide to pursue this form of treatment. However, the only way you will really know if hypnosis is right for you is by trying it.

Appendix

The answer to the nine dot problem on page 122 is:

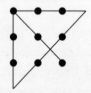

The restriction we impose on ourselves is that we want to keep the straight lines within the nine dots. No such direction is given with the puzzle and if we maintain that rule we can never solve the problem.

In much the same way we give ourselves arbitrary restrictions and hence make it very difficult to solve our own problems.

Further Reading

Brian Alman and Peter Lambron, *Self-Hypnosis: The complete manual for health and self-image*, Souvenir Press (1993)

Valerie Austin, *Self-Hypnosis*, Thorsons (1994)

Rachel Charles, *Your Mind's Eye*, Piatkus (2000)

Sheila Dainow, *Be Your Own Counsellor*, Piatkus (1997)

Eric Harrison, *How Meditation Heals*, Piatkus (2000)

Denise Linn, *Past Lives, Present Dreams*, Piatkus (1994)

Paul McKenna, *The Hypnotic World of Paul McKenna*, Faber & Faber (1993)

Brian Roet, *The Confidence to Be Yourself*, Piatkus (1998)

Cristina Stuart, *Speak for Yourself*, Piatkus (2000)

Corrine Sweet, *Overcoming Addiction*, Piatkus (1999)

Claire Weekes, *Self-help for Your Nerves*, Thorsons (1995)

Useful Addresses

Dr Brian Roet
2 The Mews, 6 Putney Common, London SW15 1HL
Tel: 020 8780 2284

British Society of Medical and Dental Hypnosis
Flat 23, Broadfield Heights, 53–59 Broadfield Avenue,
Edgware, Middlesex HA8 8PF
Tel: 020 8905 4342

BHA Hypnotherapy Association
14 Crown Street, Chorley, Lancashire PR7 1DX
Tel: 01257 262 124
Freephone: 0800 731 8443

Australian Branch of International Hypnosis Society
Rob Stanley, Administration Office, ISH,
Edward Wilson Building, Austin Hospital,
Heidelberg, Victoria 3084

Index